Also by Harley Pasternak

THE 5-FACTOR DIET

5-FACTOR FITNESS

THE 5-FACTOR WORLD DIET

THE 5-FACTOR WORLD DIET

Harley Pasternak, M.Sc.

with Laura Moser

VIKING CANADA

Published by the Penguin Group

Penguin Group (Canada), 90 Eglinton Avenue East, Suite 700, Toronto, Ontario, Canada M4P 2Y3
(a division of Pearson Canada Inc.)

Penguin Group (USA) Inc., 375 Hudson Street, New York, New York 10014, U.S.A.
Penguin Books Ltd, 80 Strand, London WC2R 0RL, England
Penguin Ireland, 25 St Stephen's Green, Dublin 2, Ireland (a division of Penguin Books Ltd)
Penguin Group (Australia), 250 Camberwell Road, Camberwell, Victoria 3124, Australia
(a division of Pearson Australia Group Pty Ltd)
Penguin Books India Pvt Ltd, 11 Community Centre, Panchsheel Park, New Delhi – 110 017, India
Penguin Group (NZ), 67 Apollo Drive, Rosedale, North Shore 0745, Auckland, New Zealand
(a division of Pearson New Zealand Ltd)
Penguin Books (South Africa) (Pty) Ltd, 24 Sturdee Avenue, Rosebank, Johannesburg 2196, South Africa

Penguin Books Ltd, Registered Offices: 80 Strand, London WC2R 0RL, England

Published in Canada by Penguin Group (Canada), a division of Pearson Canada Inc., 2010
Simultaneously published in the United States by Ballantine Books,
an imprint of The Random House Publishing Group, a division of Random House, Inc., New York

·1 2 3 4 5 6 7 8 9 10 (RRD)

Manufactured in the U.S.A.

Book design by Casey Hampton

LIBRARY AND ARCHIVES CANADA CATALOGUING IN PUBLICATION

Pasternak, Harley
5-factor world diet / Harley Pasternak.

ISBN 978-0-670-06923-1

1. Reducing diets. 2. Reducing diets—Recipes. 3. Nutrition.
I. Title. II. Title: Five factor world diet.

RM222.2.P3776 2010   613.2'5   C2009-905644-5

American Library of Congress Cataloging in Publication data available

Visit the Penguin Group (Canada) website at **www.penguin.ca**

Special and corporate bulk purchase rates available; please see
www.penguin.ca/corporatesales or call 1-800-810-3104, ext. 2477 or 2474

Contents

Introduction

In some ways, I've been researching the 5-Factor World Diet for my entire life—even if I didn't always know it. I grew up in Toronto, Canada, which the United Nations recently crowned the most ethnically diverse city in the world. More than one hundred languages and dialects are spoken in Toronto—more than in any other city in the world—and almost three-quarters of all Toronto residents are either immigrants or the children of immigrants. Like just about everyone else in my hometown, I have roots in foreign countries: my grandparents are originally from Hungary, Romania, Russia, and Poland.

Throughout my childhood, I was exposed to people from just about every culture, religion, and lifestyle you could name, and from the very beginning this diversity had a big impact on my way of looking at the world. Among other things, at a very young age I developed an insatiable appetite for a huge variety of foods, flavors, and ingredients from all over the globe. Like so many people in our international city, my family would regularly go out for Italian food, Thai food, Jamaican food,

Indian food, Portuguese food—the list goes on and on. And I was always impatient to try whatever latest exotic cuisine had come to the neighborhood.

I also spent a portion of my youth in the Caribbean, when my family lived in Jamaica, Barbados, and Trinidad, and in Miami, Florida. These early travels deepened my curiosity about different international cuisines. In Jamaica, I feasted on rice and peas and jerk chicken. In Trinidad, I enjoyed "doubles" and "buss-up shot," while in Barbados, I gorged on flying fish. In Miami, I developed a passion for Cuban food, especially black beans, plantains, and *ropa vieja,* a dish of shredded flank steak in tomato sauce. And everywhere we went, I'd taste these incredible tropical fruits that were completely unknown to most Canadians.

My family's eastern European background added yet another dimension to my perspective on international cuisine. At family meals, my grandmother served us stuffed peppers and fruit compote and *uborka salata,* a traditional Hungarian cucumber salad that was a staple in our household. The first time I went for Japanese food, my meal started with what I thought was *uborka salata*. Only afterward did I realize that it was actually *sunomono,* a traditional Japanese cucumber salad. The fact that different countries use the same or similar ingredients to produce sometimes very similar results intrigued me. I started to ask questions about the relationship between food and culture: how does what we eat reflect greater truths about how we live and what we value?

As I grew older, my zest for different flavors, smells, tastes, and ingredients grew even stronger. When I was a teenager, the Food Network was new, and it quickly became my favorite channel; I'd watch it nonstop. I was equally taken with Ming Tsai's Asian dishes, Emeril Lagasse's Cajun cuisine, and Mario Batali's Italian food. I wanted to learn it all.

Around this time, I turned into a fitness fanatic as well. I had played hockey throughout my youth and in college, and in my desire to improve my performance on the rink, I became interested in an entirely new dimension of food—not just how it tasted or how it looked and smelled, but how it could change the way *I* looked, felt, and performed.

Food wasn't just about the experience of eating, though that aspect remained incredibly important. Food was also about the results it could bring, the impact diet had on my body. The way I ate directly affected my performance as an athlete, and I saw that you could never separate diet from overall fitness.

In college, I pursued my interest in these subjects and studied kinesiology and nutrition. From early on, I really wanted to understand the scientific and technical aspects of food. In graduate school, I worked as a scientist for the Canadian Department of National Defense, conducting nutrition research. We studied the effects of different foods on soldiers' performance and energy levels.

While I was studying all these interrelated subjects, I started my personal training business in Toronto. As my reputation grew, I got the opportunity to work with a lot of Hollywood actors who were in Toronto to shoot films. To train them, I drew on my degree in exercise physiology, but I also used my degree in nutrition to help design their diets. From this convergence of experiences—my academic investigations into diet, nutrition, and physical fitness, along with my one-on-one interactions with clients—I developed what I came to call the 5-Factor Diet, a system of eating and exercising that I believe is the key to long-term health.

The basis of the 5-Factor Diet couldn't be more straightforward:

- Eat five meals a day, a practice that elevates your metabolism and stabilizes your appetite.
- Follow five specific nutritional criteria for each meal. (I go into detail about these criteria in chapter 13.)
- Build each meal around five core ingredients and take five minutes or less to prepare it.
- Work out for a minimum of twenty-five minutes five days a week.
- Enjoy one free day every week—meaning you can eat whatever you want, whenever you want.

As the 5-Factor Diet took off, so did my career. My easy-to-follow plan was garnering great results for my clients, and I soon expanded my business to Montreal and Vancouver.

With every passing month, I got the opportunity to train more actors and musicians. Since my first film, *Angel Eyes* (2001), I've been lucky enough to work with many of Hollywood's hottest, most-in-demand stars, from Halle Berry and Robert Downey, Jr., on *Gothika* to Rachel Weisz on *Constantine* and Milla Jovovich on the *Resident Evil* movies. I have toned, buffed, and fed Orlando Bloom, Jessica Simpson, Brendan Fraser, Seth Rogen, Katherine Heigl, Rob Pattinson, Hilary Duff, Miley Cyrus, and many others, getting their bodies in prime condition for films, television, and music videos.

Keeping all these celebrities in shape has allowed me to travel the world. From Singapore to Sweden, I've traveled to more than thirty countries. On many film projects, I have gone to live on location with clients to keep them in shape for the duration of the shooting. I've gone on world tours with musicians such as Kanye West, Alicia Keys, and John Mayer and spent time in such exotic places as Kuala Lumpur, Malaysia and a castle in Scotland. And wherever I've gone, I've had to rely on local resources to keep my clients fit, healthy, and looking their absolute best at all times. This necessity has made my 5-Factor Diet more expansive—and more interesting—than most other diets out there.

The scavenging aspect of my job has been particularly exciting for me in light of my longtime curiosity about international cuisines. Everywhere I go, I head straight for the food market—it is always my very first stop. (Shopping at the destination certainly seems more practical than dragging along suitcases stuffed with food!) It doesn't matter what city or country I am in, seeking out the healthiest aspects of the local cuisine is always my first priority.

Somewhere along the way, I made what seemed to be a remarkable discovery: the farther I travel from the United States, the easier it is to find foods that are both nourishing and slimming to use in my clients' meals. I also noticed that outside America—pretty much everywhere in the world, in fact—people appear to be a great deal healthier, and leaner, than they are in the States. I started to ask myself, What's going on here?

I detected a similar trend when choosing food at home. Because my day job is educating people about fitness and nutrition, my friends are always expecting me to take charge of deciding where to eat meals that are healthy and delicious. It was on one of those nights of playing the "food guide" that the idea for the 5-Factor World Diet first took distinct shape in my head.

The night started out like many others: I was tossing out suggestions for my favorite eating spots in Los Angeles. Maybe Italian? I love a good *zuppa di pesce*. Then again, you can never go wrong with the sushi at Katsuya. Or what about some churrasco chicken at that funky Brazilian place? But wait, what was I thinking? We absolutely *must* try the new Thai restaurant that everyone is raving about—I've heard great things about the lemongrass shrimp soup and chicken satay there.

As so often happens, my friends and I were soon overwhelmed by all the dining options. And then it dawned on me: without exception, every single one of the cuisines we were considering was foreign in origin. At no point did it occur to me to suggest going out for a cheeseburger and fries, a chili dog with onion rings, or a heaping plate of fried chicken and macaroni and cheese.

Sure, those typically American comfort foods taste amazing. Who doesn't love a good In-N-Out burger or Roscoe's chicken and waffles? Still, I couldn't ignore the fact that the most nutritious—and delicious— foods all come from abroad. The foods that I regularly recommend to clients and friends alike—and the foods that I myself eat most often— are almost exclusively foreign, originating in countries whose residents are thinner than we are and, not so coincidentally, live longer, healthier lives than we do in America.

Did you know that the United States has more fat people than any large-size country on the planet? In 2006, more than 74.1 percent of the U.S. population, or almost *three out of every four people* over age fifteen was considered overweight.[1] In a country with a total population of about 300 million, that means more than *225 million Americans* are at risk for hypertension, diabetes, heart disease, high cholesterol, high blood pressure, stroke, and cancer—based solely on their weight.

Conversely, did you know that people in most other countries don't have to worry so much about their health or how heavy they're getting around the middle? That's because the rest of the world doesn't have the same overwhelming issues with obesity. Other cultures and diets have somehow promoted a healthier weight than ours. But how exactly does that work? I became determined to get to the bottom of this mystery. The more questions I asked, the more I had. For example:

- Why do Japanese from the Okinawa region have one of the longest life expectancies in the world (an average of eighty-two years)? One explanation might be the practice of *hara hachi bunme,* a self-control technique that prevents them from consuming too much food.
- Why do the people of France, despite having a diet high in saturated fats and smoking obsessively, have one of the lowest rates of

cardiovascular disease in the Western world? Ingesting more phenolic compounds in their diet (commonly found in the skin of black grapes) isn't the only answer.

- How do nearly 940 million people in China stay at their ideal weight? The country's traditional plant-based diet might have something to do with it.
- Why are there even fewer overweight people in Singapore?
- Why are Italians—the people known for pizza, pasta, and cannoli—among the healthiest people in the world?
- What do the people of South Korea eat each day that causes food to move faster through their systems and keeps them lean?

In the pages that follow, I will be answering these and many other questions in great detail, and in the process revealing the diet secrets of the world's healthiest people.

Rather than focusing on what Americans are doing wrong (although I do touch on these problems briefly in chapter 1), I will be concentrating on what the rest of the world is doing right. By emphasizing what we *can* eat and what we should be doing, I hope to reframe the issue of weight management and health in a more positive light, moving more effectively toward a long-term solution that can help reshape not only our bodies but also the way we think about diet.

My experiences as a globe-trotting nutritionist and trainer have given me a unique perspective on people's eating habits around the world and what kind of impact those habits have on health. Over time, I have picked up many local tricks of the trade to make shopping for and preparing even the most exotic-sounding foods easy and fun.

In Japan, for example, a country I've visited many times with clients, I have learned that I can take them out for shabu-shabu, *robata,* or sushi. There are so many healthy ways of eating udon noodles in Japan, too. In Scotland, while touring with Kanye West, I found myself staying in a castle in the middle of nowhere. I scanned a local menu and right away stumbled upon this incredibly hearty, healthy Scotch barley soup that completely fulfilled the criteria of my 5-Factor Diet.

Over time, I began to collect international dietary secrets the way other people collect postcards or souvenir snow globes. Now, whenever I'm getting ready to return home from a trip, instead of buying a T-shirt that says "My uncle went to Moscow, and all I got was this lousy T-shirt,"

I pick up some food item that represents the place. On my last trip to Vancouver, I brought back smoked coho salmon, and on a recent trip to Finland, I filled one compartment of my suitcase with local reindeer jerky. What better way to learn about a culture than from its food?

Eventually, my investigations became more formal. After I wrote my first two books and those books were translated into other languages, I started traveling the world on book tours. There I was, by myself, with a lot more time to investigate why eating habits seemed healthier elsewhere than in the United States. Americans aren't plagued by famine; on the contrary, there's more than enough food for everybody. We have more gyms, more fat-free products, and more weight-loss infomercials than anywhere else in the world, and yet so many of us are obese and unhealthy. Why? Could it be that we're so unhealthy *because* we're so obese? If, as I believe, the answer to that question is a resounding *yes,* what exactly can we do to remedy the situation? What measures can we take to reverse these dangerous trends?

Here's where my decade of international travel comes in handy. After so many years of observing and researching other countries' dietary habits, I began the process of extracting the essence of each culture to educate people back home. My main goal in this book is to show everyone just how easy it is to live healthier. People in other countries do it all the time and without even thinking about it.

You don't have to embark on some crazy extreme diet to improve your long-term health. You just have to start making some common-sense decisions about the way you eat, move, and live. For example: Let's not deep-fry that catfish; let's broil it. Or why not make seviche instead? All you need is a lime. You don't even need any kitchen appliances. Come to think of it, you don't even need a stove.

And instead of driving down the block to the supermarket, why not put a basket on your bicycle and ride there? Or how about taking public transportation to work, even just once a week? You may be able to walk to the bus stop or train station. As you'll see repeatedly in this book, the healthiest solutions often happen to be the simplest ones as well.

My extensive travels, combined with my educational background, have clued me in on a number of secrets about nutrition, diet, and lifestyle that many foreign cultures have used for centuries. In the 5-Factor World Diet, I have devised a plan that integrates diet and lifestyle and presents specific nutritional techniques in a specific order, amplifying their fat-burning and health-boosting benefits even more than when they are used separately. This plan includes many of the most effective aspects of my 5-Factor Diet, while allowing you more creativity and flexibility than just about any diet on the market.

You will never regret embarking on the 5-Factor World Diet—the only program on the planet that combines the world's healthiest nutritional and lifestyle habits in one easy-to-follow, research-based weight-loss plan. And the best part is that you don't even need a passport to take this extraordinary journey.

PART 1

THE WAY THE WORLD
EATS AND LIVES

ONE

The World's Fattest People

Why make an effort to reform our dietary habits from the ground up? I hate to say it, but at this stage in the game, it's because we have no choice. In recent decades, we've seen a disturbing trend ripple around the world: people are getting fatter, and as a consequence, their lives are getting shorter. In 2006 there were more than 1.6 billion overweight people in the world, and the World Health Organization (WHO) projected that these numbers would grow by 40 percent by 2016.[1]

According to WHO, these are the places in the world with the most overweight adults:[2]

1. Nauru (94.5%)
2. Federated States of Micronesia (91.1%)
3. Cook Islands (90.9%)
4. Tonga (90.8%)
5. Niue (81.7%)
6. Samoa (80.4%)

  7. Palau (78.4%)
  8. Kuwait (74.2%)
  9. **United States (74.1%)**
  10. Kiribati (73.6%)
  11. Dominica (71.0%)
  12. Barbados (69.7%)
  13. Argentina and Egypt (tie) (69.4%)
  14. Malta (68.7%)

The number you see after each country reflects the percentage of adults (age fifteen and up) who have a body mass index greater than or equal to 25, which is considered overweight. Even though the United States isn't number one, experts consider it to be the most alarming country on the list. That's because with more than 225 million overweight people, the United States has the largest number of obese individuals in the world. It also exports its unhealthy habits to countries all over the globe. The passion for fast food that started in America is now a worldwide phenomenon.

According to the National Center for Health Statistics, nearly two-thirds of the U.S. population qualifies as overweight. Half of that group—or nearly one-third of the population as a whole—has been categorized as obese, which is defined as having a body mass index over 30, or more than thirty pounds over a healthy body weight.[3]

In the United States alone, obesity costs $117 billion a year, a figure that seems to get bigger every day.[4] In 1997–1999, hospital costs for obese children and adolescents topped $127 million. Just twenty years earlier, those costs were only $35 million.[5] Not only that, but our collective girth is triggering huge health problems across the board. Carrying extra weight can increase a person's risk for a wide range of conditions: hypertension, cardiovascular disease, diabetes, and some types of cancer, to name just a few. The saddest part of all is that most of the illnesses associated with obesity are 100 percent preventable.

Of course, it's not just *what* we Americans eat that keeps thickening our waistlines. It's also our misconceptions about eating in general—from how we prepare our meals to when and where we eat them. In this book, we'll be looking abroad to learn how to make more responsible, and more fun, decisions about every aspect of eating—decisions that will keep the pounds off, prolonging and enhancing the quality of our lives.

Why Are Pacific Islanders So Fat?

As the list on pages 3–4 indicates, the top seven fattest places on earth are located in the Pacific Ocean, with more than 90 percent of adults categorized as overweight in Nauru, Micronesia, the Cook Islands, and Tonga. That's nearly two times the proportion of overweight people in most developed countries.

Female Pacific Islanders have even more disproportionate weight problems, according to the International Obesity Taskforce, a group that found that more than 55 percent of Tongan women and 74 percent of Samoan women are obese.[6]

So why do these tiny island nations tip the scales to such an extent? One explanation could be that these cultures view bigness as a sign of prosperity and success. Whereas Americans and other Western countries tend to equate slimness with wealth and leisure, Pacific Islanders associate it with poverty, as Westerners did in earlier centuries.

The recent arrival of fast food might be another explanation for these alarming statistics. The too-fast Westernization of these countries' diets has wreaked havoc on Islanders' metabolism. Their bodies are simply not programmed to handle all the high-fat, high-sugar substances that people in long-industrialized nations have been gorging on for decades. And as is true all over the world, the rapid "McDonald's-ization" of a diet tends to be accompanied by rampant health problems, which is why Nauru, the fattest country on the list, also has the highest rate of adult diabetes.

Nauru's problems are particularly revealing of the factors that influence weight gain. The tiny island, with a population of thirteen thousand, has no arable land, so residents have a limited supply of fruits and vegetables (and the fruits they do have are high-sugar and low-fiber): The healthiest foods have to be imported over vast distances. Unemployment levels are also unusually high because Nauru's main industry, mining and exporting phosphates, has gone into decline.

But before we set about studying, and eventually imitating, how other cultures live and eat, we need to focus on the home front—on the bad habits that got us into all this trouble in the first place. Of all the nations on earth, we have no excuse for being this fat and unhealthy.

America is the richest nation on the planet; we have top-notch doctors, advanced medical technology, widespread food availability, and gyms on every corner. So shouldn't we be the healthiest nation in the world as well? And if so, why aren't we?

WHAT WE'RE DOING WRONG

Let's first identify the problems that we need to address in our collective lifestyle here in the United States, and in other industrialized nations— the choices that are eroding our health and shortening our lives.

Caloric Overload

To put the problem as bluntly as I can, Americans are overweight because we take in more calories than we burn. On some level, it really is that simple. WHO calls it "overnutrition," and it's a problem in many other industrialized countries as well. But Americans have a particularly egregious case of it. In 2003, the American food supply provided 3,800 daily calories for every person. That's roughly twice the Food and Drug Administration's recommended daily allowance.[7]

According to a study conducted by the Centers for Disease Control and Prevention (CDC), our caloric intake has skyrocketed since the 1970s. In 2000, women took in 22 percent more calories than they did in 1971 (1,877 calories a day in 2000 versus 1,542 in 1971). Men consumed 7 percent more (2,618 calories in 2000 versus 2,450 in 1971).[8] The figures for 2000 far exceeded the U.S. government's recommendations that women eat 1,600 and men eat 2,200 calories a day.

What might be even more troubling in the long run is that Americans are living off foods that are high in calories and artificial trans fats and precariously low in the nutrients our bodies need to thrive. High-fructose corn syrup, an all-purpose sweetener that's added to just about every packaged food you can name, is a great example of the kind of nutrient-poor, calorie-dense ingredients that have become the mainstay of the American diet. Americans also drink more sugary beverages today than at any time in history. Instead of milk and water, we are chugging gallons of high-sugar soft drinks.

All this sugar takes its toll. The U.S. Department of Agriculture (USDA) recommends that people on a 2,000-calorie daily diet eat no more than 40 grams, or about 10 teaspoons, of added sugar every day. Americans go way over the recommended amount, which is no surprise given that sugary additives can be found in packaged foods such as soups, salad dressings, ketchup, and mayonnaise—the list is endless. In many instances, these sugars are adding only one thing to our diet: calories.

Portion Distortion

We aren't just eating too much sugar; we are eating too much of everything. As the size of our portions grows, so does the size of our jeans. Meals in America seem to get bigger with every passing year, with 40-ounce drinks, heaping servings of French fries, and gigantic desserts the norm. It's no wonder that so many Americans are losing the battle of the bulge.

A study out of Rutgers University found that the portion sizes Americans eat for breakfast, lunch, and dinner have increased between 20 and 50 percent since the 1980s.[9] That means that Americans are eating 20 to 50 percent more calories at mealtime than they did just one generation ago. In restaurants, average portion sizes have doubled or even tripled over the past two decades.

You can see this "inflation" in all segments of the food industry. A Burger King burger, for example, weighed 3.9 ounces in 1954 and 4.4 ounces in 2004. (A Double Whopper weighed 12.6 ounces!)[10] At other restaurants surveyed, steaks weighed 12 ounces or more 60 percent of the time. It doesn't cost restaurants much to supersize portions, and getting twice as much food for only a few pennies more gives consumers a false sense of value (false because they will end up paying big in doctors' bills later on). Thanks to supersizing, we have grown accustomed to eating massive quantities of high-fat foods in one sitting. And sometimes we don't even bother to sit down.

To accommodate these larger portions, the size of our dinner plates also has increased in recent decades.[11] It seems that even our dishes are encouraging us to pile on the pounds.

So what's the big deal? Did you know that eating just 100 extra calories a day can add 10 pounds a year to a person's weight? Over 10 years, that's a whopping 100 pounds. To slim down as a culture, we need to start cutting our portions down to size.

Snack Happy

Snacks are another big source of additional calories. Snacking in the United States is a huge business that continues to grow every year. But snacking itself won't make you fat—if you eat the right types of snacks and the right number per day (two, according to my 5-Factor formula). The problem is that most Americans do neither. In the 5-Factor World Diet, we infuse the five-meals-a-day foundation of the 5-Factor Diet with some of the best exotic ingredients from across the globe.

On-the-Go Eating

In recent years, Americans have taken fast-food culture to an unhealthy extreme, with our famous multitasking abilities extending to mealtimes as well. Americans eat while watching TV, driving to work, even sitting in class or shopping.

No self-respecting Italian would slurp down his beloved cappuccino in the car! In many of the nations we'll be visiting, eating and drinking are not simply a means to an end, but ends in themselves. Some of the healthiest countries place a premium on eating for pleasure. Across the Mediterranean, people linger—sometimes for hours, even at lunchtime—over their meals. But fast-food chains have become more popular in some of these countries as well. According to McDonald's own website, in 2007 there were thirty-one thousand McDonald's across the globe, with more opening every year.[12]

Eating out is cheaper and more convenient than ever, but that doesn't mean it's good for you. When you aren't making your own food, you have a lot less control over what goes in it. There are no hidden ingredients in a meal you cook yourself, but you can't say the same for a meal you pick up at the drive-through.

According to a WHO report titled "The Epidemic of Overnutrition," there were 170,000 fast-food restaurants and 3 million soft-drink vending machines in the United States in 2002.[13] A survey cited in this report found that only 38 percent of all meals eaten in this country were made at home. In fact, the USDA's food intake surveys found that

Americans spend almost 50 percent of our annual food budgets on meals prepared outside the home.[14] In the 5-Factor World Diet, we will be changing that. I will be teaching you how to prepare quick, delicious, and nourishing meals in a matter of minutes. Learning how to make your own food (and figuring out what exactly goes into that food) is an essential early step toward taking charge of your overall health.

Animal Products Excess

Compared to most other nations, Americans eat through-the-roof quantities of high-fat meat two or sometimes even three times a day, seven days a week. Red meat and dairy products are beneficial in moderation, but it pays to remember that too much of a good thing can be dangerous. The steaks and hamburgers that we love so much are significantly higher in saturated fats and cholesterol than plant-based foods. Too much meat can clog our arteries and increase our risk for heart disease and other long-term health problems.

I'm not saying that you should give up meat altogether—not at all! But Americans need to learn from other countries and eat a little less of it. There are lots of low-fat sources of protein that we can start incorporating into our diet in place of our beloved rib eyes. Meat makes up just 4 percent of total calories in low-income countries, versus 13 percent in high-income countries, and America eats more meat than any other nation on earth. In 2000, the average American ate 195 pounds of red meat, poultry, and fish a year, which is 57 pounds more than people ate just half a century earlier.[15] We absolutely must work on getting that down to a much more reasonable figure.

Lazy Lifestyles

The American obesity epidemic cannot be attributed to diet alone. Americans' lives are fast-paced and high-stress to a fault. Not only do we eat on the go, without considering what we're putting into our bodies, but we also neglect other important aspects of a healthy lifestyle, such as exercise and sleep. Do you know that not getting enough rest can influence your metabolism? The Spanish do. Their insistence on squeezing in a midday nap might be one explanation for their relative slimness. And daily exercise—even if that means walking eight blocks to the grocery store every time you run out of milk—is crucial in maintaining a healthy weight. Studies have shown that we need to walk at least 10,000 steps a day to remain fit and healthy, but many Americans barely break the 3,000-step mark.[16]

This must change, because as it is, our superconvenient, sedentary culture is triggering all sorts of health issues. Compared to people in just about every other country, Americans move very little. With advances in technology, our day-to-day physical activities have taken a nosedive. A high percentage of us have cars, and we use them even for the shortest errands—driving three blocks to buy a gallon of milk, when walking the same distance wouldn't take much longer. In contrast to many European cities, our urban centers are, for the most part, built for driving instead of walking. Gas is cheaper in the United States than in Europe, and we don't have the same harsh restrictions on parking as some European cities do. As a result, we take public transportation far less frequently, which might explain why Europeans average 237 miles per year on foot and 116 miles on bicycles, while Americans get roughly one-third of that exercise, walking only 87 miles and biking 24 miles per year. And you better believe those discrepancies add up over time.

Modern jobs also don't require the same expenditure of energy that jobs once did, with manual labor severely on the decline in most major industries. The rise of various technologies (satellites, computers, wireless Internet, telephones, faxes) has made it very easy for most workers to get through the day without ever getting up from their desks—except maybe to hit the vending machine. You can buy just about anything and even do all your banking without taking a step. Although it's true that these modern conveniences make our workdays more efficient, they might be having the opposite effect on our bodies.

WHAT WE CAN DO ABOUT IT

Now that you have the basic rundown of what exactly Americans are doing wrong, you're probably asking what you can do to make improvements in your own life. Well, that's exactly the answer I propose to put forth in this book. Over the next chapters, I will be addressing each of these problems, mostly by way of contrasting Americans' increasingly unhealthy habits with those of people around the world—people who live longer and, not so coincidentally, weigh less than we do. Examining other countries' dietary and lifestyle secrets will reveal the key to keeping all of us healthy and slim through the decades.

TWO

The World's Healthiest People

Now that you have some sense of what we're doing wrong, I want to introduce you to the places where people are eating better and living longer, healthier lives. According to the CIA's *World Factbook,* these are the places that have the highest life expectancies in the world, ranked in order:[1]

1. Macau (84.36 years)
2. Andorra (82.51 years)
3. Japan (82.12 years)
4. Singapore (81.98 years)
5. San Marino (81.97 years)
6. Hong Kong (81.86 years)
7. Australia (81.63 years)
8. Canada (81.23 years)
9. France (80.98 years)
10. Sweden (80.86 years)

11. Switzerland (80.85 years)
12. Guernsey (80.77 years)
13. Israel (80.73 years)
14. Iceland (80.67 years)
15. Anguille (80.65 years)
16. Cayman Islands (80.44 years)
17. Bermuda (80.43 years)
18. New Zealand (80.36 years)
19. Italy (80.20 years)
20. Gibraltar (80.19 years)
21. Monaco (80.09 years)
22. Lichtenstein (80.06 years)
23. Spain (80.05 years)

So where, you might be asking, does the United States fall on this list? The answer is pretty grim. Despite being the richest nation on the planet, the United States comes in only at number fifty, with an average life expectancy of 78.11 years—a ranking that seems to get worse with every passing year.

In 2006, Americans' average life expectancy was 78.1 years, or 80.7 years for women and 75.4 for men, which isn't all that bad in the grand scheme of things. But even in spite of the nation's alarmingly high suicide rate, Japanese live 82.12 years on average (85.6 years for women and 78.7 years for men). In Andorra, a tiny mountainous country sandwiched between France and Spain, residents live even longer, an average of 82.51 years.

When you consider that the United States has the most money and the most advanced medical technology in the world, you might reasonably assume that Americans would also be the longest-lived people. So what do the Japanese and Andorrans know that we don't? What exactly is the problem?

I can sum up the answer in one simple word: *fat*. Research indicates that dietary habits have a direct and profound impact on health, and as we've already discussed, Americans' dietary habits are unhealthy in the extreme. More than any other factor, our expanding waistlines are to blame for our shorter life spans. That's why overhauling our lifestyle, especially our diet, is the number one change we can make to improve our health over the long term. And to make these essential changes a

reality, we need to borrow a few secrets from the countries that are getting it right.

COMBINE AND CONQUER: A SNEAK PREVIEW

What I call the combine-and-conquer strategy is an often overlooked
key to healthy eating. Variety is the spice of life, and it might also be the
secret to good health. The 5-Factor World Diet takes a global approach
to eating precisely because there are great advantages to combining multiple healthy customs from several cultures into one diet. Honestly, why
would you settle for eating one type of healthy cuisine when science and
statistics have already proved that mixing healthy cuisines together is the
key to losing even more fat, improving your health, and reducing your
risk of disease? With this diet, you don't have to.

Singapore—number four on the life expectancy list, with citizens
living almost eighty-two years on average—is a perfect example of the
power of finding the right mix of cuisines. This tiny island nation's diet
is a mixed bag in the best sense, influenced by many of its ethnically
diverse neighbors: Malaysia, China, southern India, and Indonesia.
There is even a distinct European stamp on Singaporean cuisine, since
the British founded Singapore in the early nineteenth century. Individual elements of all these cultures are still evident in Singaporean dishes
today.

You can see further proof of the benefits of the combine-and-
conquer strategy in Andorran cuisine. The average Andorran lives
more than six years longer than the average American. One reason for
this strong statistic might be that instead of eating their own distinct
cuisine, Andorrans eat a mix of different foods, combining the best
elements of the much larger regions that border their small country,
Catalonia (in Spain) and France.

By this definition, shouldn't the United States have the healthiest
food in the world? After all, few countries are home to as many different
ethnic groups. That's true, but unfortunately Americans have adopted
the *unhealthiest* elements of these groups' cuisines and blended them all
together to make one big, unhealthy soup.

By contrast, Canada, my home country—which ranks number
eight on the life expectancy list—is, like the United States, a nation of

immigrants, but with one critical difference: Canada is a salad bowl, and America is a melting pot. In a salad bowl, everything is all mixed up together, but you can still recognize each ingredient and each influence. If you pluck one out, it retains its flavor, taste, and color. In Canada, which was settled simultaneously by the French and British, ethnic influences have coexisted for centuries. Cultures meet and share influences without losing what makes each of them unique.

In the United States, everything tends to melt into one homogeneous entity. The food court in an American mall is a classic example of this phenomenon. At one food court I visited, the Chinese, Cajun, and Japanese restaurants were all giving out samples of chicken tenders. I tasted all three, and I swear to you that I couldn't tell the difference between them—not even a little bit. All three had been heavily Americanized, and they'd completely lost whatever had originally made them distinctive.

In the 5-Factor World Diet, we take a very different approach, searching the globe for the most delicious and the healthiest foods and cooking methods, then bringing them all together—but without losing what made these foods interesting in the first place. We cull the best of what the world has to offer and leave the rest behind.

Let me now explain how I ranked the world's cuisines.

WHAT WENT INTO THE RANKINGS

After nearly a decade of traveling the world with celebrity clients, exploring the best foods the world has to offer, I had a pretty good idea of which places were healthy and which were less so. But my rankings are by no means a mere matter of opinion. In addition to drawing on my own observations and experiences, I arrived at my Top 10 list based on the two groups of statistics highlighted earlier: the WHO's list of the fattest countries in the world and the *World Factbook*'s list of global life expectancy rates. There is, not surprisingly, very little overlap between these lists, since the residents of the longest-lived countries also in many cases happen to be the thinnest people in the world (with the exception of famine-ravaged countries).

Life expectancy is, of course, measured by many different statistics. In a few rare cases, a population's longevity can be attributed to having access to socialized medicine or top-notch prenatal and natal care, to lower incidences of war, or to a lower crime rate, as is the case in Iceland.

The eradication of infectious diseases in the industrialized world also has added quite a few years to the average citizen's life, which is why we focus on countries with a standard of living similar to that of the United States. The country with the shortest life span, Swaziland—whose citizens live an average of 39.4 years—is, like many of its neighbors in sub-Saharan Africa, plagued by diseases such as AIDS, poor health care, famine, lack of clean drinking water, and civil conflicts.

But again, you might be wondering why the United States, which has none of these problems, lags so far behind other countries in life expectancy and other critical measures of health. The answer is complex. For one thing, almost 47 million Americans (that's roughly the population of South Africa) have no health insurance, which means they receive little preventive care for health issues in their early stages.[2] Diabetes, heart disease, and many other problems are often neglected until far too late. The United States also has a surprisingly high infant mortality rate, with an estimated 6.8 deaths for every 1,000 live births.[3] This figure is even higher among minority populations such as Hispanics and African Americans.

When choosing the world's healthiest countries, I also looked at other statistics, including the percentage of both overweight and obese adults, how many calories the average citizen consumes on a daily basis, and the proportion of meat to vegetables in people's diet. When the data was available, I looked at how much people exercise every day and in what context. I took into account some more subjective, less easily quantifiable criteria, such as what ingredients people use, what cooking techniques are the most popular, and what, if any, impact those considerations may have on a population's health.

Confounding Factors

I want to emphasize that there are many different factors that go into the health of a nation. Although oversimplification is tempting, I made a point of taking into account what I call "confounding factors," all of which made my reading of these statistics more nuanced. So that the comparisons would be meaningful, I stuck with industrialized countries with a standard of living and an availability of resources (including food, technology, and health care) roughly comparable to those of the United States. I excluded countries that face problems such as famine and widespread disease, as in many countries in Africa, which have low obesity rates but also low life expectancies.

Genetics also plays a role that can be hard to quantify in assessing the health of any large group of people. Certain ethnic populations, for example, are more predisposed to certain health issues than others: Hispanic women are more likely to deliver preterm babies, African Americans are more vulnerable to type 2 diabetes, and people of Mediterranean descent are predisposed to thalassemia. Still other groups are more prone to certain types of cancer. I took all of these factors into account when making my list.

Lifestyle Factors

Of course, you can't judge the health of a nation just on the basis of how its inhabitants eat. You must also examine how they live—and move. With that in mind, I looked at people's physical activities in various aspects of day-to-day life and how those activities influence overall health. What occupations are most common? Do people engage in manual labor, or do they spend most of their workdays sitting in front of a computer? How widespread is technology, particularly television and other forms of stationary entertainment? How much does the average citizen walk every day? How do most people get to work—on foot, by bicycle or public transportation, or in a car—and does their mode of transportation have an impact on their health? I will be asking these questions and many others as we travel from country to country in search of better health.

Although I present a physical activity program in chapter sixteen, its framework is much more generalized than in my previous books. If you want a step-by-step workout plan, pick up one or both of my previous books, *5-Factor Fitness* and *The 5-Factor Diet,* in which I outline my program for keeping some of the biggest celebrities in the world looking their best. *The 5-Factor World Diet* has a somewhat different goal in regard to exercise: to teach you how to incorporate more physical activities into your day-to-day life.

The Big Picture

In the end, after crisscrossing the globe in search of the healthiest diets and lifestyles, I narrowed my focus to ten countries in Asia and Europe. Many of these countries' diets might be familiar to you, and that's a good thing: you may already have a grasp of the basic principles and ingredients that are key to enduring health. But be careful. Remember my trip to the food court: in many cases, we "Americanize"—that is, make more *unhealthy*—cuisines that, in their native form, could be doing us a lot of good. In this book, I'll teach you how to combine the healthiest elements of the Top 10 cuisines into a tasty, varied, and nourishing way of eating and thinking about food.

And now, what you've all been waiting for, my Top 10 list of the healthiest nations on the planet:

THE TOP 10 COUNTRIES

1. Japan
2. Singapore
3. China
4. Sweden
5. France
6. Italy
7. Spain
8. South Korea
9. Israel
10. Greece

In the country-by-country assessment in part 2, you'll find a sample of these countries' daily menus and explanations of their cuisines through the lens of five simple categories.

What They Eat

This is a broad overview of the country's diet: what types of food the people eat and why. I touch on climate, agriculture, and other factors that influence diet.

What's in It

Here I examine the ingredients that make the nation's diet unique and of interest to us, including the most popular beverages. Some of these ingredients might be familiar to you already; some of them might sound as if they came from Mars. By the time you've finished this book, I hope that all of these ingredients will have made their way into your grocery cart.

How They Prepare It

This section offers a broad look at the most common cooking methods in the country. Why do the French braise and the Chinese stir-fry? Why is baking virtually unknown to Korean chefs? I also touch on the most frequently used cooking base in each country: is it butter, olive oil, canola oil, or, as in the United States, corn oil?

How They Eat It

Here I explore the ceremonial and cultural aspects of eating. After all, it's not just *what* we eat but *how* we eat it that affects our health. This category is broad, encompassing everything from dining ceremonies to a nation's philosophical approach to food.

Occasionally under this heading, I address Americans' widespread misconceptions about certain "foreign" dishes and cuisines. Do the Chinese really begin every meal with greasy fried egg rolls? Do the Italians live off massive servings of pasta drowning in cream sauce? Sometimes it's important to examine the differences between what we *think* other cultures eat and what they actually consume.

How They Burn It

In this section, I take a look at how people burn calories. You might be surprised by how simple some of their exercise secrets are. I cover everything from formal group exercise to practical getting-to-work routines.

So let's get going. We've got a lot of territory to cover in our culinary trip around the world.

PART 2

THE 5-FACTOR WORLD DIET'S TOP 10 COUNTRIES

THREE

Japan

AVERAGE LIFE EXPECTANCY TOTAL POPULATION: 82.12 years

PERCENTAGE OF OVERWEIGHT ADULTS: 18.1 male; 27.0 female

PERCENTAGE OF OBESE ADULTS: 1.5 male; 1.8 female

MEAT CONSUMPTION PER PERSON (2002): 43.9 kg

DIET COMPOSITION (PERCENTAGE OF TOTAL NUTRIENTS):
    CARBOHYDRATES: 58
    PROTEIN: 15
    FAT: 27[1]

For many years now Japan—my 5-Factor World Diet gold medal winner—has been my go-to ethnic cuisine country of choice. It's probably my favorite place to visit for work, because I know I can always come up with a quick, easy meal for a client without too much legwork and without compromising on selection or taste.

All World Dieters should cultivate a taste for Japanese food, because it can actually prolong your life. Remember these impressive statistics: The Japanese rank number three when it comes to life expectancy, living an average of 82.12 years, according to the CIA's *World Factbook*. Not only that, but Japan's "healthy life expectancy"—a measure of how long people can feed, dress, and take care of themselves without assistance—also tops the list, at 75 years. (By contrast, Americans rank fiftieth and twenty-ninth on these lists, respectively, with an average life expectancy of 78.11 years and a healthy life expectancy of 69.3 years.) Of the 126 million people living in Japan, more than one in five is age sixty-five or older, and more than 7 million are eighty or older.[2] Not only do Japanese women live longer than anyone else on the planet, but they're also among the slimmest people: only 3 percent of Japanese women are considered obese, compared to a shocking 33 percent of U.S. women, according to the International Association for the Study of Obesity.

When you consider the astronomically high smoking rate of the Japanese—approximately 51 percent of Japanese men smoke—and their suicide rate (one of the highest in the world), these statistics are even more impressive.[3] The Japanese must have a *really* healthy diet to counteract the effects of all that nicotine and depression.

WHAT THEY EAT

The traditional Japanese diet, which is entirely different from that of almost every other culture in the world, plays a big role in these enviable statistics. The residents of the Japanese island of Okinawa—which has more centenarians (people age one hundred or older) than anywhere else on earth—eat an average of seven servings of grains daily, in addition to seven servings of vegetables and fruits and two servings of soy products. Okinawans almost never eat dairy products or meat.[4]

The rest of Japan has similarly healthy eating habits. The Japanese diet is built around rice, fish, and vegetables—foods naturally high in carbohydrates and fiber and low in calories and fat. In fact, the Japanese consume nearly 200 fewer calories a day than the average American.[5] And remarkably, despite eating so much less food, their diet is much better balanced than ours, with ingredients that contain just about every nutrient the body needs. How is that possible? Japanese nutrition guidelines suggest that people eat an average of thirty different foods every day.[6] The Japanese also get their protein primarily from fish high in omega-3 fatty acids and only rarely eat the red meat that Americans consume in such heart-stopping quantities. And instead of sugary beverages packed with empty calories, the Japanese drink mostly antioxidant-rich green tea.

Many principles of Japanese dining are universal and entirely commonsense. The Japanese place a premium on going to bed and waking up at prescribed times, as well as on eating meals at the same times every day—both routines that can help regulate metabolism and prevent overeating. And while their diet includes a broad range of vegetables and fruits all year round, the Japanese typically eat food only when it's in season. They also indulge in dessert far less frequently and in much smaller quantities than we do. Instead of cookies or ice cream, the Japanese generally end their meals with fresh fruit.

WHAT'S IN IT

Cruciferous Vegetables: The Japanese build their meals around fresh vegetables, rather than using greens as a side dish or a garnish for a big meat dish as we do. The Japanese eat cabbage and other cruciferous veggies such as broccoli, cauliflower, bok choy, and kale at just about every meal.

Cucumbers are also big in Japan. Remember that *sunomono* that bore such a close resemblance to the *uborka salata* my grandparents brought to Canada from Hungary? Other popular vegetables in Japan are ones that we would scarcely recognize, much less eat on a regular basis, including bamboo shoots, burdock, and lotus root.

Soybeans and Soy-Based Products: Packed with protein and isoflavones—which prevent everything from osteoporosis to cancer—soy is a wonderful, versatile food. Along with fish, soy—in the form of tofu, natto, and miso—provides the major source of protein in the Japanese diet. In fact, the average Okinawan eats up to 100 grams of soy each day, while the average American eats close to zero. You'll find soy in many different forms, including edamame, or boiled green soy beans, which are a popular appetizer in Japanese restaurants and a great all-around snack. Edamame are low in calories (about 40 calories per handful) and high in protein and fiber, not to mention delicious and filling.

Soba (Buckwheat Noodles): Traditional Japanese cooks make noodles out of nourishing, easy-to-digest complex carbohydrates such as buckwheat. Despite its name, buckwheat has no relation to wheat, which makes it a safe alternative for anyone avoiding gluten (found in wheat, oats, rye, and barley). In fact, like quinoa, buckwheat isn't even a grain—it's a seed related to rhubarb and sorrel.

The health benefits of buckwheat are staggering. It's a rich source of fiber, magnesium, and all eight essential amino acids. Buckwheat also contains an antioxidant called rutin, a flavonoid that can lower your risk of developing high cholesterol and high blood pressure, as well as D-chiro-inositol, which drives carbohydrates into your muscles without raising insulin levels.

Buckwheat flour is the key ingredient in a number of different cultures' traditional dishes. French galettes, Russian bliny, and Ukrainian *hrechanyky* are all buckwheat-based dishes. Kasha, or roasted buckwheat groats, is a common eastern European breakfast or side dish. In Japan, buckwheat flour is most often used to make soba noodles, the Japanese answer to spaghetti. The Japanese incorporate soba noodles into a range of different dishes, both hot (as in a vegetable broth) and cold (as in a salad). These delicious, nourishing noodles are increasingly popular in the United States as well, and you can buy them in most midsize grocery stores across the country.

Shirataki: Shirataki is another fantastic alternative to traditional starchy pastas. These noodles are made out of a variety of root vegetables (most of which are native to Asia) and occasionally have tofu added for a smoother texture. They are extremely low-carb—and extremely delicious! The Japanese eat other noodles, too, including harusame, e-fu, bifun, and cellophane noodles (made from mung bean starch). If you see any of these noodles on a menu, why not give them a try?

Fish High in Omega-3 Fatty Acids: Fish, the cornerstone of the Japanese diet, is a much healthier source of protein than the red meat that's the staple of the American diet. It's lower-fat, and oily fish such as salmon, tuna, herring, and mackerel (a Japanese favorite) are rich in omega-3s, which are essential for good cardiovascular health. Fish oil can also increase your mental alertness and even help combat depression. Fish is a great source of selenium and iodine as well. Be sure to choose the lower-mercury fish, which I list on page 107.

Sushi, and its rice-free counterpart sashimi, are probably the most quintessentially Japanese foods there are. People love sushi for the simplicity and beauty of its presentation. Void of heavy sauces, oils, and seasonings, sushi also contains no added fats and happens to be extremely low in calories. Although it's mild-flavored, sushi comes in so many different forms—from nigiri to hand rolls to maki—that you couldn't possibly get sick of it. It's filling, too—what more could you ask of a food?

Seaweed: Japan is an island, so it's only logical that the Japanese would regularly feast on seaweed and other sea vegetables. Lucky for them, seaweed is rich in iodine and other health-boosting minerals and microelements. It's also an excellent source of fiber. And, best of all, seaweed tastes delicious, adding a rich, savory flavor to a wide variety of foods. Try sprinkling it on salads or adding it to soups. Of the many different types of seaweed, nori and kombu are the most popular varieties in Japan.

Nori: This mild-flavored, cold-water seaweed is most often processed into the thin sheets used to wrap sushi rolls. The Japanese also eat nori on its own as a snack. You can try toasting this versatile seaweed and crumbling it over soups, salads, and veggies.

Kombu: This large, warm-water kelp is the seaweed used to flavor miso soup. Some Japanese chefs treat kombu as we would a bay leaf, adding it to rice or a stew during cooking, then discarding it before serving. You can also add kombu to a marinade for meat, fish, or vegetables.

Wakame: This is a kelp that looks and tastes like spinach lasagna. It's similar to kombu and can be used in many of the same ways, particularly in soups and salads and as a topping for other dishes. I use a lot of wakame in my recipes. Soak dried wakame in water, and it will expand to about ten times its size. To serve as a vegetable, cut out the central vein after soaking, then simmer for 10 minutes. Or cut into small pieces and serve in a salad. Because of its kelp content, wakame is rich in protein, calcium, iodine, magnesium, iron, and folate. Kelp also is rich in lignans, which may provide protection against certain cancers. Lower rates of breast cancer have been reported in Japanese women who eat a diet high in kelp.

Hijiki: This brown seaweed grows wild on the rocky coast of Japan. It's a traditional food that has been used as part of a balanced diet in Japan for centuries. Hijiki is known to be rich in dietary fiber and essential minerals such as calcium, iron, and magnesium. According to Japanese folklore,

> ### Beverage of Choice: Green Tea
>
> The choice of beverage in Japan is another reason the Japanese diet tends to be much lower in sugar than ours. Rather than reach for a supersize soda loaded with sugar and calories, the Japanese favor heart-healthy, antioxidant-rich green tea, which has been shown to fight certain cancers, ease pain, and even burn calories. Kombucha, a sweet tea made with the kombucha mushroom, is another Japanese favorite. This drink has become increasingly popular and available in the United States.

hijiki aids health and beauty, and the thick, lustrous hair of the Japanese people is connected to their regular consumption of small amounts of hijiki. The Japanese usually eat hijiki with other foods, such as vegetables or fish. It may be added to soups or foods that have been steamed, boiled, marinated in soy sauce or fish sauce, or cooked in oil. Hijiki may also be mixed in with rice for sushi, but it is not used as a wrap to prepare sushi.

Mushrooms: About half of the World Diet countries have a favorite food in common: mushrooms. These yummy fungi consist mostly of water and therefore have very few calories. They also provide a wide range of nutrients, such as potassium and selenium, which can protect cells from free radicals in the environment. Shiitake mushrooms, which are used in all sorts of Japanese dishes, have even been used to fight cold and flu symptoms.

HOW THEY PREPARE IT

Boiling: The Japanese boil the staple of their diet, white rice, with edamame, spinach, mushrooms, and other vegetables.

Grilling: Grilled fish is common in Japan. Cooking meat and vegetables on a hibachi (the Japanese equivalent of a barbecue pit) is another treasured tradition. Yakitori—bits of grilled chicken served on a stick, shish kebab style—is a popular street food in Japan.

Robata is another traditional Japanese grilling method that says a

---

Cooking Oil of Choice: Sesame, Soybean, or Canola

Though many of their dishes, like sushi and sashimi, are made without any oil at all, the Japanese do use sesame, canola, or soybean oil in their cooking.

---

great deal about Japanese cuisine in general. Basically, all the ingredients are grilled right in front of you, then laid out with no adornment at all: no sauces, no spices or strong seasonings, no oils, nothing but clean, healthy food, grilled to perfection. The flavor of the food—whatever it might be, a fresh vegetable or a slab of fish—is unobscured and pure. On my first visit to a *robata* house in Tokyo, I remember thinking, *I never knew what red snapper tasted like before!*

Steaming: The Japanese steam rice, fish, clams, and tofu. Steamed buns, with either salty or sweet fillings, are another staple food.

Serving Raw: Sushi and sashimi are the most famous foods the Japanese eat raw, but they also enjoy a wide selection of salads and raw vegetables.

Deep-Frying: Tempura is about the only big category of Japanese food that's fried. To make tempura, vegetables or seafood is lightly coated with batter and fried. The Japanese occasionally fry tofu as well.

HOW THEY EAT IT

It isn't just the ingredients or the cooking methods that have kept the Japanese healthy to such an advanced age; it's the way they eat their food, too. Over the centuries, they've developed a series of dietary guidelines—some practical, some philosophical—to keep them slim and spry.

They know when to say when.

One explanation for Japan's ranking as number 163 on the list of the world's fattest countries is *hara hachi bunme,* the practice of eating until just about 80 percent full. Instead of going for seconds or dessert right away, the Japanese are taught to wait twenty to thirty minutes after reaching this 80 percent threshold. More likely than not, their bodies will no longer crave any additional food.

"Eat like a crane" is a popular regional proverb in Japan (and Korea as well).[7] The narrow shape of a crane's beak means that the bird can only pick at its food; wolfing down a tremendous amount all at once is not, anatomically speaking, an option.

The next time you sit down to eat, try to practice a little *hara hachi bunme* and "eat like a crane." Chew your food thoroughly, as the Japanese do, and stop before you're full. Eat slowly and deliberately. As you begin to feel full, put down your fork and let your body digest what you've just eaten.

They believe that presentation is everything.

Mingei, the union of form and function, is a core principle of Japanese culture that extends to their relationship with food. The Japanese do not view food merely as nourishment. It's also a satisfying, sensual pleasure— a truth that's too often lost in Americans' frenzied, drive-through lives.

In Japan, a good meal should stimulate all five senses, including sight. Think about the beautiful burst of color inside a sushi roll: a perfect testimony to the pride that Japanese chefs have always taken in the visual presentation of their food and a concept that we have pretty much lost in North America. When you're in a food court, your senses are assaulted by a mishmash of sights and sounds and smells, but when you're in a Japanese restaurant, the décor tends to be minimalist, which allows you to focus all your attention on the food in front of you. You can approach your meal with a clear palate and a clear mind. Pausing to enjoy the beauty of your food may also help you slow down to savor every bite. And as we know, eating slower generally translates to eating less.

An extension of *mingei* is the Japanese concept of *goshiki,* which states that every meal should have at least five colors: white (rice, tofu, fish); yellow (scrambled eggs, squash); red or orange (carrots, sweet potatoes); green (any green vegetable); and black, dark purple, or brown (eggplant, seaweed). *Goshiki* ensures that a meal will please both the eyes and the palate—not to mention fulfill most nutritional requirements. The Japanese also strive to incorporate different cooking techniques into every meal. A typical bento lunch might include a boiled egg, fried rice, grilled vegetables, steamed salmon, and fresh fruit.

They separate their meals into distinct courses.

Part of the caloric control in Japanese food stems from the limited use of added fats in dishes such as sushi and tofu, but the moderate portions also play a big role. One way the Japanese limit portion size is by serving each course on a small, decorative dish or by using one plate divided into distinct compartments, as in the bento box. The Japanese make a point of enjoying each distinct flavor on its own.

This long-standing Japanese custom is another example of *mingei,* the marriage of form and function. Instead of heaping an entire meal onto a single massive plate, the Japanese devote an individual plate or bowl to each component. If the dish happens to be small, the amount of food put on it also will be small. Studies have shown that larger plates encourage larger portions and lead to the consumption of more total calories per meal.

This tradition not only limits portion size and promotes the Japanese ethos of food as a source of beauty and pleasure, but also serves to lengthen the duration of meals. Because even the tiniest course is given its own dish or compartment, the Japanese have developed the habit of eating small bits of food over a long period of time—pecking away slowly, just like a crane.

**They treat red meat as an occasional side dish,
not a main course.**

Meat rarely plays a starring role in Japan. Vegetables, noodles, and rice have that honor. The liberal use of soy (primarily tofu) and heart-healthy fish instead of meat also keeps saturated fat levels low in traditional Japanese fare.

HOW THEY BURN IT

In previous centuries, the Japanese had a more active lifestyle than they do today. As more residents drive cars and take sedentary office jobs, the average Japanese weight is steadily creeping up. Still, to a much greater extent than Americans, the Japanese have a more active life. For the business of everyday life, they travel almost everywhere on foot. Tokyo is famous for its advanced subway system, and the vast majority of residents walk from their homes to the nearest subway stop. A recent study found that people who use "active transportation" (which means they have to walk to public transportation hubs) burn five to nine pounds of additional fat every year, compared to just two pounds in the United States, where we drive everywhere.[8]

More formal fitness activities have also made inroads into Japanese life. The Japanese corporate culture encourages good health and physical fitness, both of which have been shown to boost productivity during business hours.

DAILY MENU

Breakfast: A healthy Japanese breakfast might consist of steamed rice, miso, and either grilled fish, a small omelet, or a seaweed salad. Miso soup is a popular breakfast dish. This broth-based soup generally contains nutrient-packed tofu or soba noodles in addition to seaweed, and its high water content keeps the calories low. Another popular Japanese breakfast is *chawanmushi,* which literally means "steamed in an egg bowl." *Chawanmushi,* an egg custard dish, is also eaten at lunch and dinner.

Lunch: A typical hot lunch might feature a rice or noodle bowl with fish or meat, or a frittata-like dish called *okonomiyaki*. For a cold lunch on the go, a Japanese might bring a bento box containing rice balls, a sushi roll, and an assortment of pickled vegetables.

Dinner: Dinner, the main meal of the day in Japan, is usually built around the same ingredients used at breakfast and lunch. It might feature *robata*— freshly grilled meat, vegetables, or fish with no added oils or seasonings. Another healthy option would be a dish of cold soba noodles with a side of sushi. To finish the meal, Japanese might have a cup of hot green tea.

TO-GO TIPS

- Elevate your enjoyment of your meals (and limit portion sizes) by putting a big emphasis on presentation.

How We Misinterpret It

Restaurants serving sushi and sashimi are becoming increasingly popular across the United States, even in small towns, but Americans tend to add local touches that are none too healthy, serving sushi rolls filled with cream cheese, for example, or mayonnaise—not exactly typical Japanese ingredients. American Japanese restaurants also serve a disproportionate amount of the unhealthiest item on the traditional Japanese menu, tempura. And the U.S. interpretation of chicken teriyaki is often overly salty.

- Break up your meal into separate courses to slow down your dining experience.
- Try to eat a wide variety of foods every day—the fresher, the better.
- Add more seaweed, fish, and soy to your diet.

FOUR

Singapore

AVERAGE LIFE EXPECTANCY TOTAL POPULATION: 81.98 years

PERCENTAGE OF OVERWEIGHT ADULTS: 22.0 male; 23.8 female

PERCENTAGE OF OBESE ADULTS: 1.8 male; 1.3 female

MEAT CONSUMPTION PER PERSON (2002): 71.1 kg

I have already mentioned Singapore as a country with a diet and lifestyle that Americans should try to emulate. Ranked fourth on the list of countries with the longest life expectancy, with citizens living an envi-able 81.98 years on average, Singapore also has a notable ranking on the list of the world's fattest countries: it comes in at number 162, with only an estimated 22.9 percent of the population considered overweight. While Singapore's excellent health-care system, extensive public walk-ing paths, and several government-run fitness programs have played some part in these statistics, the country's diet is also a huge factor.

WHAT THEY EAT

What *don't* Singaporeans eat? A trading port since the British colonized it in the nineteenth century, tiny Singapore has one of the most diverse cultures—and cuisines—in the world. Singaporeans serve up the ultimate fusion food, influenced by Malaysian, Chinese, Indian, Thai, and British cuisine. Without a doubt, from a culinary perspective Singapore is the most interesting place I have ever visited.

The island of Singapore is located due south of China, between Malaysia and Indonesia. The Philippines, Cambodia, and India, are all relatively nearby. Singapore's location at the crossroads of so many otherwise dissimilar nations has made it a natural melting pot of foods and cultures from all over Asia, as well as Britain. The food modern Singaporeans eat bears the imprint of all the nationalities that have had an impact on the island over the past two centuries. You might have a Chinese porridge (congee) for breakfast, a traditional *rojak* for lunch, and a Thai curry for dinner. Anything goes in this multicultural nation.

WHAT'S IN IT

Rice: Like other Asian countries, Singaporeans pair rice with just about every other item on the menu. They usually eat this staple carbohydrate three times a day. It's served boiled or fried, or sometimes even cooked in coconut milk or with saffron and ghee (clarified butter). Singaporeans also eat several different types of noodles, such as rice vermicelli and yellow egg noodles. Malaysian rice cakes are another common food.

Fish: Like so many of the healthiest people in the world, Singaporeans consume a wide selection of fresh fish. Fish head curry is a typical Singaporean red snapper dish that represents a fusion of Chinese and Indian cooking styles. Singaporeans also frequently eat spicy chili crab and black pepper crab.

Tropical Fruits: Because Singapore is situated right on the equator, the island offers a rich profusion of tropical fruits, which are often eaten instead of dessert. The durian, which locals call "the king of fruits," is probably the most famous fruit native to the island. The rambutan and

---

Beverage of Choice: Coffee or Tea

Not so surprisingly given the "anything goes" nature of food on the island, Singaporeans have a taste for both coffee (like Westerners) and tea (like their Asian neighbors). They often add sweetened condensed milk to both beverages—not a habit I recommend adopting unless you strictly follow all the other Singaporean dietary protocols as well.

---

mangosteen are among the many other tropical fruits frequently eaten in Singapore.

Poultry: Singaporeans eat chicken in the Indian style, cooked in a tandoor (clay oven), or the Indonesian style, cooked in a spicy broth. They also eat duck in a variety of Chinese preparations.

Spices: Nothing shows the multicultural influences on Singaporean cuisine like the spices its chefs use: the strong flavors are what make Singaporean cuisine stand out. Chiles are one of the most prominent spicy borrowings from Malaysia; tamarind, curry, and turmeric show the influence of India.

HOW THEY PREPARE IT

Stir-Frying: Like Chinese chefs to the north, Singaporeans lightly stir-fry many main dishes, especially meat and vegetables. Also as in China, they usually pair these stir-fries with rice or noodles.

Grilling: Kebabs and other forms of grilled meat have become popular in Singapore.

HOW THEY EAT IT

Street food "hawkers" are the most popular alternative to home cooking in Singapore. "Hawker centers"—Singapore's version of the American food court—serve up some of the tastiest street food on the island, with Malaysian vendors positioned right next to those specializing in south-

> ### Cooking Oil of Choice: Canola or Sesame
>
> Like other Asian countries, Singaporeans primarily cook with heart-healthy canola or sesame oil. Butter (like other dairy products) is generally scarce.

ern Indian, Chinese, and Indonesian food. Because food purchased from hawkers tends to be relatively inexpensive, Singaporeans of every income bracket eat at these centers on a regular basis.

HOW THEY BURN IT

Singapore is a compact, highly urbanized city-island with excellent public transportation. As a new country, it has an amazing infrastructure and great urban planning, so there are wonderful trails for running, walking, and biking all over the city. The trails are beautiful and welcoming around the clock. Singapore is such a densely populated, efficiently built city that everything is either within walking distance or within reach of public transportation. It's very easy to go without a car there.

Because so many expatriates from the United States, Europe, and Asia live in Singapore, gyms are also popular. Government-run fitness programs have increased the population's awareness of the importance of daily exercise. In 1993, the prime minister of Singapore officially launched a national program called the Great Singapore Workout, a low-impact aerobic routine set to local music.

Yoga is popular as well, further proof of the Indian influence on everyday life. It will not elevate your heart rate high enough or for long enough to burn a significant amount of calories, but it's nevertheless great for improving balance, increasing flexibility, and relieving stress.

DAILY MENU

Breakfast: Congee, a type of Chinese porridge, is a common breakfast choice in Singapore, as is *kaya,* a sweet coconut-egg jam, served on toast. *Roti prata,* based on an Indian dish, is also popular for breakfast.

Lunch: A Chinese-style soup of stir-fried noodles, vegetables, and pork is one lunch option. Others include a plate of curried chicken noodles or some Indonesian-style rice noodles in a coconut curry served with shrimp.

One of the most common everyday foods in Singapore is *rojak,* a traditional Indonesian or Malaysian dish that has been interpreted many times over by Singapore's food hawkers. *Rojak*—a Malay word meaning "wild mix"—comes in both sweet and savory varieties and consists of either fruits or vegetables combined with fried soybean cakes and fried dough, then sprinkled with peanuts and dressed in a sauce of fermented prawn paste, sugar, tamarind, lime juice, and powdered red chiles. No single food could better represent Singapore's amazingly diverse culinary roots.

Dinner: Dinner in Singapore might consist of chicken grilled in an Indian tandoor and served with chapati, a typical Indian flatbread. Singaporeans also might dine on Indonesian *nasi padang,* which is steamed rice combined with any number of vegetables and proteins. Another common choice, and as typically Singaporean as *rojak,* is *laksa,* a spicy noodle soup (made with either coconut milk or fish broth, depending on the type) that synthesizes elements of Chinese and Malaysian cooking. Dessert might be red bean soup, green bean soup, mango pudding, or watermelon balls—all relatively low-sugar meal closers.

TO-GO TIPS

- Take a multicultural approach toward eating. Mix up flavors and influences.
- Spice up your food to keep things interesting.
- Take advantage of your city's public transportation possibilities, as well as any bike paths or walking trails in your area.
- Experiment with some exotic fruits.

FIVE

China

AVERAGE LIFE EXPECTANCY TOTAL POPULATION: 73.47 years

PERCENTAGE OF OVERWEIGHT ADULTS: 24.7 male; 33.1 female

PERCENTAGE OF OBESE ADULTS: 1.8 male; 1.6 female

MEAT CONSUMPTION PER PERSON (2002): 52.4 kg

DIET COMPOSITION (PERCENTAGE OF TOTAL NUTRIENTS):
   CARBOHYDRATES: 60
   PROTEIN: 12
   FAT: 28

China might be a massive nation, but its individual citizens certainly aren't. In fact, China comes in at an impressively low number 148 on the WHO's list of the fattest countries, with only 28.9 percent of the population considered overweight. Life expectancy varies greatly in the different regions of China. Although the average life expectancy of a Chinese mainlander is only 73 years, residents of two major Chinese cities, Hong Kong and Macau, live longer than almost anyone else on earth. People in Macau, who top the list of global life expectancy rates, live an eye-popping 84.36 years on average, while Hong Kongers live 81.86 years.

Up in Smoke?

The Chinese diet makes up for some other lifestyle shortcomings. Roughly 67 percent of urban males smoke regularly and altogether more than 300 million Chinese smoke. That's more people than live in the entire United States! The Chinese smoke more than any other people on the planet, and smoking contributes to four out of the five leading causes of death in the country.[1]

It's no coincidence that Macau and Hong Kong are very different culturally from the rest of China, too. Macau was under Portuguese rule for more than four hundred years, while Hong Kong belonged to Britan from 1842 to 1997. Taiwan, which has an average life expectancy of almost 78 years, has also been a beneficiary of foreign influences. Over the centuries, the small island, which lies across the Taiwan Strait from mainland China, was colonized by the Spanish, then the Dutch, then the Japanese. Only after World War II did the Chinese Nationalist government take control of Taiwan once and for all.

Although the cuisines of Macau, Hong Kong, and Taiwan still bear the stamp of visitors from abroad, the predominant food is uniquely Chinese, and these cuisines rank among the healthiest in the world.

WHAT THEY EAT

When I say "Chinese food," the image that might immediately come to mind is of a glistening platter of sweet-and-sour pork from the take-out place down the street, or maybe those miniature fried egg rolls that leave your fingertips greasy but taste oh so delicious. I want you to put those beloved dishes out of your mind for the time being, because the traditional Chinese diet has almost nothing in common with the high-fat, MSG-laden Chinese food that's so popular in the United States.

The core of the traditional Chinese diet can be summed up pretty easily: plants, plants, and more plants. The Chinese build their meals around fresh seasonal vegetables, fruits, whole grains, and beans. These nutritious ingredients generally make up at least two-thirds of the average Chinese meal, which is what accounts for the fact that the Chinese eat more than three times as much fiber as we do.[2] I cannot emphasize enough how important this is. Fiber is one of the most important components of a healthy diet (see chapter 13), and North Americans simply don't get enough of it. Fiber can slow down digestion (this is a good thing!), stabilize blood sugar levels, lower cholesterol, and reduce the risk of developing diabetes and some cancers.

Another big benefit of the plant-based diet of the rural Chinese is that it's naturally rich in disease-fighting antioxidants and plant-based nutrients called phytochemicals. As a result, heart disease is rare in China. Whereas the average Chinese has a blood cholesterol level of 127, the U.S. average is closer to 215.[3]

The traditional Chinese diet is also good for your waistline. Somehow, even though Chinese people consume more calories per pound of body weight than we do, they have a much lower incidence of obesity. How'd they pull that off? One explanation is the low fat content of the traditional Chinese diet. According to a book called *The China Study,* rural Chinese derive 6 to 24 percent of their calories from fat. By contrast, the American diet consists of 35 to 40 percent fat.[4]

The virtual absence of meat in Chinese cuisine helps keep the fat content low. For economic reasons, Chinese chefs typically add only the smallest shavings of meat to their dishes. Meat acts as a garnish to add flavor to an entrée; it is almost never a stand-alone course as it is in U.S. Chinese restaurants. In fact, meat makes up only an astounding 2 percent of the traditional Chinese diet.

WHAT'S IN IT

Chinese Leafy Greens: The green vegetables indigenous to China break all nutritional records. Chinese (napa) cabbage and bok choy (the word *choy* means "leafy green" in Chinese) are not only high in fiber but rich in nutrients such as beta-carotene, vitamin C, and iron. These veggies taste great stir-fried or steamed, which is how the Chinese typically prepare them. Chinese broccoli and mustard greens—which are similar, but not identical, to their U.S. counterparts—are also great options.

Other Vegetables: Daikon, a versatile root vegetable, is incorporated into a wide variety of Chinese dishes. Bamboo shoots, Chinese mushrooms,

Beverage of Choice: Oolong Tea

Tea is an ancient beverage, discovered more than five thousand years ago in China. According to legend, in 2737 B.C. the emperor Shen Nung—known as "the Divine Healer"—was sipping boiling water when the wind carried a few tea leaves into his pot. This accident of history changed Chinese culture forever. Today, more than six thousand varieties of tea are available in China, which is still the largest tea producer in the world. The Chinese drink their favorite beverage, which is 99 percent water and naturally zero-calories, with meals and throughout the day. Syrupy, high-calorie soft drinks are a relatively recent innovation in China and utterly foreign to rural Chinese.

Although Chinese drink all types of tea, oolong is the mainstay of the Chinese diet. Called the "champagne of teas," oolong is generally darker than green tea and lighter than black tea. Oolong is rich in polyphenols and catechins, antioxidants that are renowned for their anti-inflammatory qualities. Drinking oolong tea regularly can help lower cholesterol, regulate blood sugar, and possibly even fight cancer. Oolong tea has also been shown to decrease stress, aid digestion, and help detoxify the body of smoke, alcohol, and other toxins. A recent study found that oolong tea also can increase metabolism by 10 percent for two hours after drinking it.

Tea still ranks among the most popular beverages in the world, second only to water. About half of all Americans regularly drink tea, 85 percent of which comes iced (and all too often sweetened as well). Most of this tea (about 83 percent) is black.[5] Black tea also contains polyphenols and has weight-loss benefits, but it has more caffeine than oolong and green varieties.

and snow peas are used in many Chinese stir-fries. In general, the Chinese see vegetables as main dishes, not merely as accompaniments to meat.

Soybeans: Like other Asians, the Chinese eat soy products in many different forms. Tofu and soy sauce, both key components of the Chinese diet, can be a great source of vegetable protein.

> **Cooking Oil of Choice: Corn, Soybean, Canola, or Peanut**
>
> Vegetable oil (corn, soybean, or peanut) is a foundation of Chinese cooking. Traditionally, the Chinese have added oil only sparingly when preparing food, but recently this has changed. Over the past twenty years, the per capita annual consumption of vegetable oil has skyrocketed, and peoples's weights are increasing as a result.

White Rice: Instead of white bread, the staple carbohydrate of the Chinese diet is white rice. Although white rice does make your blood sugar spike, especially compared to the more nutritious brown and wild varieties, it is still healthier than the white bread that Americans often eat many times a day.

Garlic and Ginger: These disease-fighting herbs make an appearance at just about every meal in China.

HOW THEY PREPARE IT

Stir-Frying: Stir-frying meats and vegetables in a wok is great for preserving water-soluble vitamins such as A and C. A wok is a must-have item in Chinese cooking. You can prepare just about any food—rice, vegetables, meat, fish, edamame, tofu—without using too much oil. With a wok, you can just braise or flash-cook veggies without overcooking them. Slightly crunchy veggies have more nutrients, and they taste better, too. Stir-frying gives food all the flavor of deep-frying, with only a fraction of the fat.

Steaming: Next to stir-frying, steaming is the most popular cooking method in Chinese cooking. Steaming is also one of the gentlest ways to prepare meat and vegetables, preserving nutrients and flavor.

Red Stewing: Red stewing is the process of cooking food in soy sauce and water, instead of just water alone (which is the Western idea of stewing). The Chinese use this method—which adds both flavor and color to dishes—to prepare pork, beef, ham, chicken, duck, and other meat.

Adding Flavor with Healthy Sauces

Sauces make an appearance in nearly every stage of Chinese cooking. They're used for marinating, stir-frying, and dipping. Most Chinese sauces—oyster, hoisin, black bean—are soybean based. Ginger is another core sauce ingredient. It has a delicious tangy flavor and has also been shown to soothe an upset stomach.

- **Oyster Sauce:** This thick, dark brown sauce is a key ingredient in many Chinese stir-fries. Traditionally, Chinese cooks made oyster sauce by boiling fresh oysters, then seasoning them with soy sauce, salt, and spices. Today, most oyster sauces in America have nothing whatsoever to do with oysters. Instead, they are "oyster flavored," with a high content of sugar, cornstarch, MSG, and caramel coloring. Some even include sodium benzoate as a preservative. These mass-produced sauces have zero protein and tons of sodium. See chapter 14 for tips on finding healthier, more authentic sauces.

- **Hoisin Sauce:** The Chinese equivalent of our barbecue sauce is made from ground soybeans mashed together with garlic, chiles, salt, and other spices.

- **Black Bean Sauce:** Sauces made from boiled black soybeans—the oldest known soy-based food—are common in Cantonese cooking. Orange peel, ginger, and five-spice powder are often added to the sauce for extra flavor.

Deep-Frying: I would be lying if I said that the Chinese never under any circumstances deep-fry their foods. They do, but only occasionally—by no means as often as American interpretations of Chinese food might lead you to believe.

HOW THEY EAT IT

They philosophize about their food.

There's a traditional Cantonese saying: "Eating is as important as the sky." Often in China, food and philosophy go hand in hand. Many aspects of food are infused with the country's ancient philosophical traditions.

Accordingly, the Chinese take the concept of a "balanced" meal to new levels. I'm not just talking about combining protein and carbs here. A cornerstone of Chinese philosophy is yin and yang, which states that all opposing forces in the universe are interdependent. According to this view, most problems in life, from a domestic disturbance to a massive thunderstorm, result from an imbalance of yin and yang.

So it makes sense that in China, foods don't just have flavors. They also have specific energetic properties, dominated either by yin (feminine, passive, cool) or yang (masculine, active, hot). Most vegetables, for example, are considered yin foods, while most animal products and grains are considered yang. When preparing a meal, Chinese cooks try to balance the yin and yang of the foods, as well as their colors, flavors, and textures. This emphasis on balance extends to all aspects of the meal. A food from the sea is typically paired with a food from the land, just as yin vegetables are paired with yang whole grains.

The Five Elements Theory

The five elements theory is an extension of the yin and yang principle and a perfect complement to my 5-Factor World Diet principles. An ancient Chinese medical text recommends "five grains for nutrition, five fruits, five meats for benefit, five plants for fullness."

The number five also informs the five elements theory of Chinese cooking—yet another example of the link the Chinese see between a person's diet and his or her physical and spiritual well-being. According to Chinese philosophy, all matter in the universe is composed of five elements (also referred to as the five phases or five forces): fire, earth, metal, water, and wood. There are also five flavors—bitter, sweet, spicy, salty, and sour—and five major organs—heart, spleen, lungs, kidneys, and gallbladder. The wood element corresponds to the gallbladder and sour flavors; earth to the spleen and sweet flavors; metal to the lungs and spicy flavors; water to the kidneys and salty flavors; and fire to the heart and bitter flavors.

To keep the five elements in balance, the Chinese recommend eating all five flavors at every meal. A properly balanced meal also contains five colors: red, yellow, white, blue, and green.

Even cooking methods reflect this philosophy. Stir-frying is considered a yang technique, and so yin vegetables are often prepared in this manner. Similarly, garlic, chiles, and ginger—all yang foods—work well at countering the yin of vegetables.

Mixing different types of foods and cooking methods is an important part of Chinese cooking. Individual ingredients don't matter as much as the combination of elements united in a given meal.

They slow down the pace with chopsticks.

The Chinese invented chopsticks and still eat most of their meals with them today. Using chopsticks—especially if you're not used to them—can be a great technique for slowing down a meal. Chopsticks prevent diners from taking overly large bites. Despite their name, chopsticks are not designed to chop. That's why Chinese food is traditionally prepared in small, bite-size pieces—just enough to fit between the two slim sticks.

The Chinese use spoons for soups and occasionally forks as well, but one thing you'll almost never see at a Chinese table is a knife. Again, there's a philosophical reason behind this dining practice. Because the knife could be used as a weapon, it has the potential to disrupt the peace and harmony of a meal and is therefore banned from the table.

They skip dessert.

Although Americans think of fortune cookies as the typical Chinese meal ender, these cookies actually originated in Japan and appeared in California in the early twentieth century. In fact, fortune cookies weren't produced in China until 1993! The Hong Kong entrepreneur who started importing them to China in the late 1980s advertised them as "genuine American fortune cookies."[6]

Dessert in general is a foreign concept to most Chinese. Instead of rich, dairy-based pies, cakes, and cookies, Chinese usually polish off their meals with a bowl of soup, especially red bean soup. According to traditional Chinese medicine, excessively sweet foods can weaken the spleen and hamper digestion. Fruit is a less common alternative, since it's often a main-course ingredient in Chinese cooking. Some Chinese also like to end a meal with sunflower seeds.

The Snack That's a Meal: Dim Sum

Snacking has been part of Chinese culture for a very long time. The Chinese tea ceremony—known as dim sum, which translates as "touch the heart"—came into being when travelers on the ancient Silk Road needed to stop for refreshment but didn't want to spoil their appetites for dinner.

Tea is the most important component of dim sum, which consists of a series of small dishes. Steamed dumplings and buns, pot stickers, and rice noodle rolls are among the most popular dim sum dishes. All of these dishes were created to give travelers energy to continue the journey through central Asia. In recent years, most Chinese grocery stores have started offering microwavable, fast-food versions of these traditional afternoon snacks.

HOW THEY BURN IT

Every morning, right before dawn, millions of Chinese gather in public parks all over the country and exercise together. One of the most popular early-morning activities is tai chi, which began as a martial art.

The tai chi symbol is the yin and yang, and the word *chi* means "energy" in Chinese. The purpose of tai chi is to break up energy blockages in the body. Once this chi is released, it flows through the body and opens up energy channels, which leads to better digestion, a stronger respiratory system, and a body capable of healing itself.

A series of gentle, flowing exercises that often seem to be performed in slow motion, tai chi promotes balance, concentration, and stability. After a typical tai chi workout, you probably won't be very sweaty, but you will feel calm and centered. Just as the Chinese believe that you don't eat simply to fill your belly, they also believe that you don't work out simply to tone your booty. Tai chi does build muscle tone, however, while also promoting inner relaxation and focus. Another benefit: you can learn tai chi at any age. In fact, in China the majority of the sport's practitioners are elderly.

Another traditional Chinese form of exercise is qigong. (The *qi* comes from the same Chinese word as the *chi* in *tai chi*.) Qigong uses aerobic and breathing methods to release pent-up energy in the body.

How We Misinterpret It

The boundaries between traditional Chinese cuisine and Americanized Chinese cuisine have become increasingly blurry in recent years, as the urban Chinese adopt a diet that looks more and more like ours. But Americans also broadly misinterpret the food they call "Chinese" in this country.

In 2004, there were more than thirty-six thousand Chinese restaurants in the United States. Chinese food has become our national ethnic food of choice. But from the very beginning, Chinese food in America has been a hodgepodge of Chinese and American tastes. When the first Chinese restaurants sprang up during the California gold rush, they catered to both Chinese and American laborers.

A report by the Washington-based Center for Science in the Public Interest found that traditional heart-healthy Chinese cuisine is the last thing you'll find in many North American Chinese restaurants. Our versions of Chinese dishes tend to be battered, deep-fried, and sugary sweet. Consider that a dinner-size order of lemon chicken packs 1,400 calories, 13 grams of cholesterol-raising saturated fat, and 1,700 milligrams of sodium because of the deep-fried breading and salty sauce. That's a caloric load equivalent to three McDonald's McChicken sandwiches plus a 32-ounce nondiet soft drink. An order of orange crispy beef—a dish of flour-coated, deep-fried meat—has 1,500 calories, 11 grams of saturated fat, and 3,100 milligrams of sodium. Even the vegetable dishes studied were surprisingly high in added fat and salt. An order of stir-fried greens was found to deliver 900 calories and 2,200 milligrams of sodium; eggplant in garlic sauce weighed in at 1,000 calories and 2,000 milligrams of sodium.

Here's the scoop on some of Americans' favorite "Chinese" dishes.

- **Chow mein**—crispy-fried egg noodles served with vegetables and meat—is an extremely popular "Chinese" dish in the United States. It was actually invented here, in the mid-1800s, by Chinese immigrants working on the transcontinental railroad. The Chinese have their own version of chow mein, but it's much less oily than what we find in the States. For instance, the noodles in China are lightly stir-fried rather than deep-fried to a crisp. It's no wonder that a single serving of beef chow mein at P. F. Chang's has 770 calories and 24 grams of fat!

- **Chop suey** is another "Chinese" dish that originated in the United States. One legend claims that Chinese chefs in New York invented this dish in honor of Chinese ambassador Li Hung Chang's visit to America in 1896. Another claims that chop suey (which translates literally as "little pieces") was another product of the California gold rush around 1849. Typically made from bits of bamboo shoots, celery, onion, water chestnuts, bean sprouts, and some sort of meat, chop suey is served over rice and cooked with a salty, cornstarch-laden gravy that is virtually unknown in China. Although chop suey might be a bastardized version of *tsap seui*, a stir-fried dish from Toisan, a rural town south of Canton and the ancestral home of many nineteenth-century immigrants to the United States, it would be hard to find a meal in rural China as bad for you as a dish of American-made pork chop suey, which might have as much as 680 calories and 50 grams of fat.

- **Crab rangoon and pot stickers** are foods born in California. It's no coincidence that people refer to these "Chinese" dishes as "fried ravioli."

What else do the Chinese do to stay fit? They walk everywhere. Until relatively recently, very few Chinese owned cars, so most conducted the daily business of life on foot.

DAILY MENU

Breakfast: Soup, or watery porridge (sometimes called congee), is a component of almost every meal in China. The Chinese also eat leftovers from other meals, such as rice and pickled vegetables, for breakfast.

Lunch: Lunch in China tends to be pretty simple, perhaps a bowl of hot noodles, vegetables, and a few scraps of meat in broth. Dim sum is also a popular lunch choice. Busy urban Chinese on the go might pick up a quick lunch from a street vendor. When I was in Beijing, I passed through a mall-like network of street vendors selling every kind of lean protein you can imagine, including octopus, lean pork, and tiny fish.

Dinner: Dinner is typically the most elaborate meal of the day in China. The main meal might include tofu with cabbage; fried rice with onions, garlic, and vegetables; stir-fried rice with vegetables and tofu skin (yuba); or a whole steamed fish flavored with garlic and ginger and served with rice.

TO-GO TIPS

- Use chopsticks to slow down your meal.
- Adopt a philosophical approach toward your food: think before you eat.
- Build your meals around fresh local vegetables.
- Think of meat as a garnish, not a main course.
- Try replacing soda and calorie-dense coffee drinks with green tea.

SIX

Sweden

AVERAGE LIFE EXPECTANCY TOTAL POPULATION: 80.86 years

PERCENTAGE OF OVERWEIGHT ADULTS: 44.9 male; 54.5 female

PERCENTAGE OF OBESE ADULTS: 11.0 male; 11.8 female

MEAT CONSUMPTION PER PERSON (2002): 76.1 kg

DIET COMPOSITION (PERCENTAGE OF TOTAL NUTRIENTS):
CARBOHYDRATES: 51
PROTEIN: 14
FAT: 35

Swedes aren't just blond and beautiful—they also have the tenth-highest life expectancy in the world, according to the CIA's *World Factbook*. Although the Swedish health-care system certainly plays a role in the robust health of this Scandinavian people (government-run health care covers nearly 85 percent of all medical bills nationwide), the Swedes also have an enviably healthy lifestyle and diet.[1] Only 27 percent of Swedes are considered overweight, and fewer than 12 percent are obese, although these numbers have increased in the past decade.

WHAT THEY EAT

Traditionally, Swedish cuisine tends to be rustic, hearty, and practical, more economical than elaborate. That said, the Swedish kitchen has always been very receptive to culinary influences from abroad. In the seventeenth and eighteenth centuries, French food had an effect on traditional Swedish cooking, and today the average Swede dines not only on local pickled herring but also on sushi, kebabs, and falafel. Because of the long Swedish winters, the Swedes structure their year-round diet around dairy products such as yogurt and milk, dark fibrous breads, and fish, fish, fish.

WHAT'S IN IT

Cabbage: Although fresh vegetables can be hard to come by in Sweden's cold climate, Swedes do eat a lot of winter vegetables such as cabbage. Cucumbers also make frequent appearances at the Swedish table. Preserved vegetables are common, and root vegetables, especially potatoes, are served with most meals.

Dairy Products: Swedes drink a great deal of milk—in fact, only the Finns drink more—and have a high calcium intake. Calcium can help the body switch from a fat-storing to a fat-burning mode, keeping you slim. Both children and adults often have a glass of milk with their meals, making it the standard mealtime beverage for all generations.

Dark Bread: Swedes eat bread often, but they favor dark bread such as rye or pumpernickel, which is much healthier than the refined white bread Americans usually eat. Swedish bread often has added fiber in the form of bran or oats.

Berries: Although fresh fruits are relatively scarce in Sweden, blueberries and strawberries are all over the menu, bottled in jams and served fresh as dessert. Blueberries have anti-inflammatory and antioxidant qualities that are useful in fighting disease and slowing the aging process.

Fish: Much of Sweden is surrounded by water, so it makes sense that Swedes eat lots of heart-healthy oily fish such as salmon and herring.

Gravlax, or cured salmon, is eaten on crisp flatbreads throughout the day. Smoked eel, trout, whitefish, and crayfish are also popular staples.

One of my all-time favorite meals in Sweden was lunch at the Avalon Hotel in Göteborg, where the waiter served me a plate of herring prepared five different (and all equally delicious) ways, with a side of high-fiber, low-calorie cabbage. I remember being impressed and not a little astonished that the chef could do so much with such a simple fish.

Potatoes: Because potatoes grow year-round in even the most inhospitable climates, Swedes eat them in great quantities. Lunch and dinner are rarely served without a side dish of potatoes.

HOW THEY PREPARE IT

Curing and Smoking: The Swedes cure fish so that it lasts for many months. Smoking fish helps keep fresh catches tasty longer. Both curing and smoking are great for preserving healthy foods through the winter, when nature might not provide fresh provisions.

Pickling: The Swedes pickle many foods to preserve them through the long winter. Fermented (or pickled) foods contain digestive-system-friendly probiotics.

Boiling: The Swedes boil most vegetables. Although boiling might not be the tastiest way to prepare a food, it gets the job done without adding any fat.

Cooking Oil of Choice: Margarine

Sweden is the only World Diet country where margarine, instead of oil, is frequently used in cooking. Swedes consume much more margarine than butter—almost twice the amount.

HOW THEY EAT IT

They practice *lagom*.

In Swedish, *lagom* means "just enough," a principle often applied at mealtime. Swedes eat until they are satisfied but not full.

They take the tops off their sandwiches.

The traditional Scandinavian way of making a sandwich involves only one piece of bread. The typical open-faced sandwich puts more emphasis on the vegetable and fish fillers and less on the bread.

They prize variety.

Just as Swedes like to eat foods from all over the world, they also like to eat numerous dishes at one meal. The smorgasbord is a Swedish invention, and on holidays Swedes choose from a wide selection of dishes, both hot and cold, served buffet style on a large table.

HOW THEY BURN IT

Year-round physical fitness is a key component of Swedish slimness. Whatever the outdoor temperature (and it is often very cold), Swedes manage to stay fit. They love the great outdoors, even in subzero temperatures. Nordic walking, which began in Finland, has become a craze in Sweden, too. It involves walking with long poles, which helps build core muscles. Every step burns 20 percent more calories than walking without the poles. Almost half of all adult Swedes belong to some sort of sports organization or fitness club. Last but not least, because gasoline is so expensive in Sweden, many people walk or bike to work.

DAILY MENU

Breakfast: A Swede might begin the day with porridge, fermented milk or yogurt, or some form of pickled fish. A special-occasion breakfast might include lingenberry (Swedish cornberry) pancakes.

Lunch: Swedes often eat a full, cooked lunch perhaps consisting of boiled new potatoes or potato pancakes, pickled herring, and pea soup. They also might have cabbage rolls or a root vegetable soup, especially in winter.

Dinner: For dinner, a Swede might enjoy a hearty meal of traditional Swedish meatballs, or, depending on the season, filling pork-and-potato dumplings or a lighter dish of crayfish.

Snack: Swedes generally have a small snack, such as an open-faced sandwich or a piece of fruit, between meals.

TO-GO TIPS

- Go outside and exercise, regardless of the temperature. Make working out a way of life.
- Make the most of your area's natural resources, even if you live in a cold climate.
- Cut back on the bread content of your sandwiches. Removing the top is an easy way to halve your bread intake.
- Eat until you've had just enough, not until you're stuffed.
- Dairy is good! Stick to low-fat or nonfat versions. If you have a dairy intolerance, try lactose-free products.

SEVEN

France

AVERAGE LIFE EXPECTANCY TOTAL POPULATION: 80.98 years

PERCENTAGE OF OVERWEIGHT ADULTS: 34.7 male; 45.6 female

PERCENTAGE OF OBESE ADULTS: 6.6 male; 7.8 female

MEAT CONSUMPTION PER PERSON (2002): 101.1 kg

DIET COMPOSITION (PERCENTAGE OF TOTAL NUTRIENTS):
  CARBOHYDRATES: 47
  PROTEIN: 14
  FAT: 39

Buttery croissants, foie gras, gooey cheeses, full-fat yogurts, rich pastries and chocolates, wine with dinner every evening—how do the French seemingly indulge in every bad-for-you food under the sun and still stay so slender?

Remarkably, despite the astronomical fat content of their foods, the French have much lower obesity rates than Americans: 9.5 percent compared to our 33 percent. They also have a pretty impressive life expectancy: 77.7 years for men and 84.2 years for women. Although certain outside influences contribute to these enviable stats—including the

French health-care system, consistently rated among the best in the world—the French also have a few secrets to staying thin and healthy.

WHAT THEY EAT

The French take great pride in their national joie de vivre—taking pleasure in the finer things in life, especially food. There are no prohibited foods in French cooking, whatever the fat content. In fact, the French eat anything and everything they want—in moderation. The emphasis on quality over quantity is a cornerstone of the French culinary philosophy. They prefer to fill up on small quantities of heavy foods rather than stuff themselves with empty calories, so even if the ingredients are high-fat, the portions are consistently small. Fat-free or low-fat "diet" foods are anathema to everything the French hold dear about dining.

For the French, the bottom line is, eat whatever you want—just make sure you enjoy it. Treat every meal like a special event, a little break from the humdrum. The French seldom snack, as they would rather save their appetites for the main event. The French attitude toward wine is similar. Although they enjoy red wine—which has been shown to lower the risk of cardiovascular disease—just about every evening, they tend to drink wine only with their meals, and rarely to excess.

WHAT'S IN IT

Eggs: The French make omelets for casual dinners at home and often eat hard-boiled eggs with mayonnaise as a side dish at lunch. Eggs also are incorporated into hollandaise and other sauces.

Leeks: Leeks, which are related to onions and garlic (also big ingredients in French cuisine), are used to make vichyssoise and other dishes. The French prize leeks not only for their taste but also for their diuretic properties. Shallots make frequent appearances in French cuisine as well.

Other Vegetables: A typical French main course consists of a meat dish accompanied by two side dishes of vegetables. Zucchini, eggplant, green peas, asparagus, haricots verts (thin green beans), carrots, potatoes, and a variety of mushrooms are among the many options a French chef might choose from. Since most French people buy their vegetables at open-air

> **Beverage of Choice: Water**
>
> The French are famous for drinking red wine, but there's another tradi-
> tional beverage that also keeps them fit and healthy: water. Serving
> mineral water with meals is common in France, and hydrating while
> eating is a good strategy for filling up faster.

markets, the selection really depends on the season. Salads play a regular
role in France. They are generally served after the meal and might
include endives or fennel.

Yogurt: The French love their dairy products (and that includes butter),
often consuming plain yogurt after a meal in lieu of dessert. Yogurt is a
source of active probiotic cultures—the "good" bacteria our immune
system needs to stay healthy. Like milk, yogurt is high in calcium, vitamins B_{12} and B_2, potassium, and magnesium. Although low-fat and
nonfat dairy products have made inroads into French cuisine in recent
years, the French prefer good old-fashioned full-fat yogurt and milk.
The key, as in everything else about French eating, is portion control.
For the French, the main consideration is quantity, not fat content.

Mussels: The French are fond of all sorts of seafood—from calamari to
trout to canned sardines. But no one dish typifies the French emphasis
on freshness and simplicity like *moules marinières,* a simple preparation
of mussels with garlic, onions, parsley, and white wine.

Herbs and Spices: The French are known for their subtle flavorings.
The most common seasonings in French cuisine are rosemary, tarragon,
marjoram, sage, and thyme. A "greatest hits" of French seasonings is
herbes de Provence, a mixture of herbs such as rosemary, marjoram, basil,
bay leaf, thyme, and lavender. You can find it in most grocery stores.
Fleur de sel is a famous French sea salt used throughout the country.

Meat and Poultry: A big meat dish is often the centerpiece of the main
meal of the day in France: foie gras, chicken, beef, lamb—whatever happens to show up on the plate (and it could be just about anything). But
even though some of these are rather fatty meats, they usually account

> ### Cooking Oil of Choice: Butter
>
> The French aren't afraid of cooking with full-fat, artery-clogging butter instead of oil. Their fearlessness goes along perfectly with their anti-dieting ethos: eat whatever you want, provided it's in moderation. Although they do cook with butter every day, they aren't likely to eat gobs of it on one chunk of bread after another before dinner is even served.

for a small portion of the meal, and there will always be several side dishes accompanying them.

HOW THEY PREPARE IT

The French take great pride in the art of cookery and tolerate no shortcuts. In addition to the following cooking techniques, broiling, grilling, and the very advanced flambéing are commonly used in the French kitchen.

Baking and Roasting: The French use the dry heat of an oven to prepare a number of meat dishes. They roast meat uncovered at high temperatures, reducing the heat gradually as the meat cooks.

Braising: The French cook many foods in liquids that have been flavored with wine, meat stock, or vegetable juices. This adds nuance and depth without adding unnecessary fat.

French-Frying: The French do fry foods, but not in the deep oil that we might associate with "French fries." Instead, they shallow-fry in a skillet, usually using olive oil or another oil that is low in saturated fat. Because they never fry in lard or oils that are high in saturated fat, the French version of frying actually bears a closer resemblance to sautéing.

HOW THEY EAT IT

They have a healthy attitude toward food.

So how can the French indulge in such heavy foods and still stay so slim and heart-healthy? According to Mireille Guiliano, author of *French*

Women Don't Get Fat: The Secret of Eating for Pleasure, it all boils down to the French attitude toward food. The French eat for pleasure and only in moderation.

The French believe that deprivation leads to imbalance and an unhealthy preoccupation with food. Instead of starving themselves one day and pigging out the next, they eat small portions of a wide range of foods 365 days a year. They also shun "fake" diet foods, preferring small quantities of high-fat foods over massive quantities of low-fat (but not zero-calorie) foods.

They structure their meals.

To prolong the pleasure of dining, the French break up their meals into multiple courses. Dinner often consists of four courses and spans two or three hours, and families still dine together as regularly as they did fifty years ago. A typical dinner consists of a starter (perhaps raw vegetables, or crudités), a main course, a salad, a cheese course, and a little dessert. The French also make a point of eating at a nicely laid table (instead of on a TV tray), with a tablecloth, cloth napkins, and real china.

This emphasis on structure and ceremony also applies to the timing of meals in France. People try to eat at roughly the same times every day, and they discourage any activity that threatens to spoil the pleasure of their meals.

They eat at a slow pace.

Despite the explosion of fast-food chains in France over the past several decades, the French still believe that food should be enjoyed while sitting at a table and without any distractions. (Most French cars don't have cup holders, because the French believe it's a sacrilege to drink coffee while driving!) So despite the sky-high fat content of many French meals, their slow, deliberate dining methods often mean that they consume fewer calories than Americans do. For me, the pace of their meal exemplifies all that is good about French cuisine. I will never forget a breakfast I had one summer in Juan-les-Pins, in the south of France. The entire breakfast consisted of café au lait, a toasted baguette, brie, and some jam— which took me nearly two and a half hours to consume! Instead of wolfing down the food, I focused on people-watching, reading, and soaking up the sun. It was among the most enjoyable meals of my life. And despite the decadence of the food I was eating, my caloric intake per minute was much lower than in an average American breakfast.

They indulge, but always in moderation.

Quality over quantity is the name of the game. Portion sizes in U.S. restaurants are much larger than those in French restaurants, according to one study that compared restaurants in Paris and Philadelphia. And buffets, especially of the all-you-can-eat variety, are virtually unknown in Paris. In French homes, too, people eat smaller portions of richer foods.

HOW THEY BURN IT

Inefficiencies built into everyday life— such as shopping for groceries on the way home from work every day, as the French do—can actually make you healthier in the long run. Walking to the market every day will ensure that you get at least some exercise. This tradition also helps keep fattening snack foods out of reach when those midnight cravings strike. The French shop when they are out of food; they do not load the pantry for several months at a time. Because they shop so frequently, the French buy plenty of fresh fruits, vegetables, and other perishables. And they try not to shop when hungry. Also, as in many of the 5-Factor World Diet countries, the French are less dependent on their cars than Americans are. They walk, cycle, or take public transportation to conduct much of their daily business.

DAILY MENU

Breakfast: For breakfast, a typical French person might have a brioche or croissant with butter or jam and a café au lait or hot chocolate.

Lunch: In a study that tracked the eating habits of fifty blue-collar workers in Paris and Boston, the French participants consumed 60 percent of their day's calories before 2:00 P.M.[1] On weekends and special occasions, the French might have an elaborate, multicourse dinner; the rest of the time, lunch is the most important meal of the day. On a busy weekday, a French person might eat a simple lunch of *salade niçoise* with onion soup, ratatouille, or a ham, cheese, and tomato sandwich on a toasted baguette. Mineral water is usually the only beverage the French drink at lunchtime.

Dinner: During the week, dinner tends to be light and easy to digest. On special occasions, it's broken up into several distinct courses. It might start with a bowl of onion soup, followed by a main course of coq au vin with haricots verts and new potatoes. A green salad is generally served after the main course. The meal might end with a cheese plate and/or dessert.

TO-GO TIPS

- Choose your meals carefully and eat at roughly the same times every day.
- Prize quality over quantity. Worry less about the content of your meals than about how much you eat. Everything in moderation is the French key to success.
- Do your daily errands on foot.
- Buy foods as you need them, keeping your focus on fresh and seasonal foods. Eat a wide variety of local fruits and vegetables throughout the year.
- Savor the moment, from the flavors, aromas, and aesthetics of your meals to the company you dine with. Take your time and enjoy!

EIGHT

Italy

AVERAGE LIFE EXPECTANCY TOTAL POPULATION: 80.20 years

PERCENTAGE OF OVERWEIGHT ADULTS: 38.3 male; 52.7 female

PERCENTAGE OF OBESE ADULTS: 12.6 male; 12.9 female

MEAT CONSUMPTION PER PERSON (2002): 90.4 kg

DIET COMPOSITION (PERCENTAGE OF TOTAL NUTRIENTS):
   CARBOHYDRATES: 51
   PROTEIN: 13
   FAT: 36

According to a 2007 report by the World Health Organization, men in the mountains of northern Italy enjoy the longest life expectancy in the world, with an average life span in excess of 80 years—that's a full five years longer than the average American male lives. Italians also have a relatively low obesity rate, with only 10.2 percent of the population considered obese in 2006 (although this figure was up from 7 percent in 1994).[1]

WHAT THEY EAT

How do Italians stay in such tip-top condition while gorging themselves on enormous plates of pasta and greasy pepperoni pizzas? The answer is, they don't. Italian food is one of the most popular ethnic cuisines in the United States, but what most Americans consider "typical" Italian food bears little resemblance to Italian food in its native setting. Pizza, ravioli, lasagna, spaghetti and meatballs, fettuccine Alfredo—some of the most popular "Italian" dishes in the United States—have been Americanized beyond recognition.

Like other cuisines in the Mediterranean region, the traditional Italian diet is rich in fruits and vegetables, grains, beans, nuts, seeds, lean protein (fish and poultry), a small amount of dairy, and a little wine. Italians place a premium on fresh, local foods and straightforward, uncomplicated flavors. And like the inhabitants of neighboring countries, Italians get most of their fat from healthy, unsaturated sources such as olive oil, not the through-the-roof quantities of meat and cheese that play a starring role in many American Italian dishes.

Yes, the Italians love their pasta, but they almost never eat it as a main course. It's usually served on a very small dish between the salad and meat courses. What's more, the sauces served over Italian pasta dishes have little in common with the goopy cream or heavy-duty meat sauces we find on pasta here. Instead, pasta sauces in Italy tend to be tomato and vegetable based. And while pizza in the United States is often served on a thick crust and piled high with cheese, pizza in southern Italy, where it is most prevalent, generally consists of a thin whole-grain crust topped with tomatoes and vegetables and just a sprinkling of cheese.

WHAT'S IN IT

Tomatoes: The Italians consume more tomatoes than any other people in the world, but they generally don't purchase ready-made tomato sauces. Italian tomato sauces—like most elements of Italian cooking—are simple and fresh, a concentrated source of the many nutrients tomatoes have to offer.

Tomatoes are rich in vitamins A, C, and K, and they're also one of the few dietary sources of lycopene, a powerful antioxidant that's been

---

When in Rome

When I think of "typical Italian fare," I inevitably remember a dinner I once had while working on the southeastern Italian coast at Brindisi. The entire meal consisted of a single simple, light dish, *zuppa di pesce,* a traditional peasant soup made with various seafood in a flavorful broth, poured over some stale bread. It contained clams, oysters, mussels, sea bass, squid, shrimp, and other fish caught off the coast. I cannot begin to describe how enjoyable that meal was. When I left the table, I was full—in both stomach and spirit.

---

proved to protect cells from oxygen damage and reduce the risk of cardiovascular disease. Lycopene helps fight nearly all forms of cancer, including colorectal, prostate, breast, endometrial, lung, and pancreatic. Cooked tomatoes provide more lycopene than raw ones, and virgin olive oil, garlic, and basil—the three essential supporting ingredients in a basic marinara sauce—can enhance the absorption of lycopene.

Pasta: Contrary to popular belief, pasta can be incredibly healthy, especially when it is homemade. It's a source of thiamine, folic acid, iron, riboflavin, and niacin. Just be careful how much of it you eat and what you put on it. The Italians eat pasta in small quantities, as a side dish.

Oregano and Basil: For flavor minus the fat—and numerous health-boosting properties—Italians infuse their dishes with a variety of subtle herbs and spices, especially basil and oregano. These herbs are packed with antioxidants. In addition, oregano contains thymol and carvacrol, two antimicrobial agents that reduce infection. Basil, the main flavor in pesto, contains flavonoids, which protect cells and chromosomes from radiation and oxygen-based damage.

Balsamic Vinegar: The best balsamic vinegar in the world is made in Modena, in northern Italy, and Italians throughout the country use it to add a touch of sweetness without extra calories to dishes. Balsamic vinegar also has some important health benefits. It can help suppress your appetite, can encourage the production of metabolism-boosting digestive enzymes, and might even strengthen your bones.

Beverage of Choice: Espresso

Millions of Italians rely on a morning espresso. Because of the way it is made, an espresso might contain two to three times the amount of healthy antioxidants as coffee made with other brewing methods. And unlike a Frappuccino from Starbucks, which might contain as many as 800 calories (that's as many calories as in three McDonald's hamburgers!), an espresso has no calories at all.[2] Espresso comes in many different varieties, from the regular espresso to the macchiato to the cappuccino and finally the latte, depending on the amount of milk. An espresso has no milk at all, and the latte is chock-full of it. Espresso also has less than one-third the caffeine of regular American coffee, so you can have more than one a day.

Italians also regularly drink a single glass of a local red wine and a glass of sparkling water with dinner.

Legumes: Beans and legumes—especially cannellini beans (white kidney beans), green beans, and chickpeas—are staples of traditional Italian cuisine, used in soups, salads, pasta dishes, and risottos. Beans are a virtually fat-free source of protein, soluble fiber, iron, and B vitamins.

Artichokes: The artichoke is an extremely versatile vegetable that can be stuffed, steamed, or turned into a delicious sauce—not just dipped in melted butter the way Americans enjoy it. Artichokes are high in magnesium, folic acid, fiber, and vitamin C.

Lemons: Lemons are used in all sorts of dishes in southern Italy, where they grow in abundance. Italian cooks also use them in salad dressings and squeeze them over meat and fish to add flavor. Lemons are high in vitamin C, which is essential to maintaining a strong immune system.

Fruit: A small bowl of *fighi e albicocche* (figs and apricots) is a common dessert in Italy. Southern Italians frequently end their meals with a fresh, delicious lemon ice. Soda, candy, and other junk food have only made their mark on Italian culture in recent years.

> **Cooking Oil of Choice: Olive**
>
> Italians consume a great deal of olive oil, which can lower cholesterol and protect against heart disease. But though olive oil is a relatively healthy source of unsaturated fat, it's calorically dense, and Italians are careful not to overdo it. At American Italian restaurants, the waiter will often bring out a little dish of olive oil for you to dunk your bread in. This practice is much less common in Italy.

HOW THEY PREPARE IT

Grilling and poaching are the most common ways to prepare foods in Italy. Like so much else about Italian cuisine, these cooking techniques are straightforward and healthy. Sautéing, baking, and steaming are also common.

HOW THEY EAT IT

They savor la dolce vita.

Italians take pleasure in la dolce vita—literally, "the sweet life"—which contributes to their health and longevity. Americans may think of Italian dining as indulgent and heavy, but this is a misconception. In fact, Italians have only one large meal a week, and that's usually Sunday lunch. The rest of the week, Italians *do* linger over their meals, but not because the food keeps on coming.

Italians like their meals to last a long time, often extending relatively small meals into three or even four separate courses. They may go for a stroll both before and after a meal, enjoying the fresh air and drawing out the pleasure of the meal for as long as possible. Why rush the pleasure of the dining ritual, one of the greatest enjoyments life has to offer?

Did you know that this slow approach to eating might do more than enhance their enjoyment of life? It might also benefit their waistlines. A recent Japanese study published in the *British Medical Journal* found that eating quickly until full can more than triple a person's risk of becoming overweight.[3]

Long meals are just one aspect of Italians' famously low-stress lifestyle. They rarely work more than forty hours a week, and they have one of the longest vacation allotments in Europe.

They have a weekly "free day."

From Monday through Saturday, Italians generally eat modest portions of healthy foods. Sunday is their national "free day," the one day of the week when they indulge in massive, filling meals. It's no coincidence that Sunday lunch is also the longest meal of the week, sometimes lasting up to five hours.

The rest of the week, Italians stick to small portions, often served in multiple courses. They also eat a small snack between breakfast and lunch. This keeps their blood sugar levels relatively steady and discourages bingeing.

Italians tend to load up on salad and go light on pasta. In Italy, pasta is usually a small course between the salad and the main dish. Most often it's served in a light tomato sauce or a little olive oil. Italians also eat salad as often as twice a day. By filling up on greens at the beginning of a meal, they are less likely to pig out when the pasta course arrives.

They pass on cooking traditions from one generation to the next.

Eating is an intergenerational affair in Italy. At a typical Sunday lunch, grandparents, parents, and children all eat together. But it's not just the sit-down portion of the meal that involves the whole family; it's also the preparation. Passing cooking techniques from one generation to the next is the logical extension of the Italian emphasis on food and family. Small children learn firsthand how to cook by spending time in the kitchen with their parents and grandparents.

HOW THEY BURN IT

Before and after the dinner hour, you will see Italians strolling leisurely through town, stopping to chat with neighbors and look in store windows. Grandmothers walk with their grandsons, husbands with their wives. This tradition, known as the *passeggiata,* is a classic illustration of

---

How We Misinterpret It

Chicken Parmesan is a perfect example of an artery-clogging "Italian" specialty that was actually born in the United States. This dish of breaded and fried chicken cutlets drenched in marinara sauce and melted mozzarella reputedly first saw the light of day in New York or New Jersey in the 1930s, the invention of Italian immigrants from Naples. But don't expect to find chicken Parmesan on a menu in Italy. At least two key features of the dish—the combination of meat and tomato sauce and the massive amount of mozzarella—would be utterly unfamiliar to most Italians.

---

the Italian art of taking pleasure in life. These relaxing nightly ambles are first and foremost social events, but they're also a wonderful way to facilitate digestion and get in a bit of gentle exercise before bed.

Another fat-burning habit practiced all over Italy is walking to the market. Rather than drive to the grocery store and load up on a week's worth of supplies, Italians typically walk to their local markets and buy what's freshest, letting the best-looking veggies dictate the evening menu. Remember, convenience is not a priority. Italians generally look down on frozen and precooked meals.

Finally, like many other Europeans, Italians are soccer mad. From a very young age, Italian children are on the soccer field, and they continue to play through adolescence. In many cases, their passion for playing this high-impact sport endures into adulthood.

DAILY MENU

Breakfast: Breakfast in Italy is usually pretty simple, consisting of espresso and either cereal, a small roll, or a small dish of yogurt.

11:00 A.M. Snack: This often consists of a cappuccino (espresso with milk, *never* cream or half-and-half), yogurt, or fruit. It's important to note that although Italians typically have a midmorning snack, they never snack after dinner. They believe that food should be digested before they go to bed.

Lunch: Lunch is generally broken down into two small courses, such as a small plate of pasta followed by a small piece of fish or chicken and vegetables.

Dinner: Traditionally the largest meal of the day, dinner is served relatively early in the evening (by European standards, that is) to allow proper digestion before bed. To prolong the pleasure of dining, Italians extend the meal over several courses: a small salad, pasta with a tomato or vegetable sauce, a small portion of fish or meat, vegetables, and fruit for dessert.

TO-GO TIPS

- Start your day with a jolt of espresso.
- Take time over meals: savor the ceremony. Eating should be an art and a pleasure.
- Load up on healthy whole grains and fresh local veggies.
- Take a walk before and after dinner.
- Indulge in a weekly "free day." After six days of discipline, you're allowed to splurge on Sunday!

NINE

Spain

AVERAGE LIFE EXPECTANCY TOTAL POPULATION: 80.05 years

PERCENTAGE OF OVERWEIGHT ADULTS: 47.8 male; 55.8 female

PERCENTAGE OF OBESE ADULTS: 15.8 male; 15.6 female

MEAT CONSUMPTION PER PERSON (2002): 118.6 kg

DIET COMPOSITION (PERCENTAGE OF TOTAL NUTRIENTS):
CARBOHYDRATES: 47
PROTEIN: 14
FAT: 39

Spain lies at the crossroads of many different cultures. In ancient times, it was populated by Greeks, Romans, Hebrews, and North Africans. Today, Spain's diverse culinary traditions reflect the country's long multicultural history: the Spanish have been practicing the combine-and-conquer technique for centuries now!

Despite all the rich, indulgent foods the Spanish eat (think manchego cheese and cured pork), they are a remarkably slim people: the Spanish obesity rate hovers around 15 percent. They are also among the longest-lived people on earth.

WHAT THEY EAT

Although the Spanish never skimp on high-fat foods or wine, their diet revolves around healthy basics native to the area: citrus fruits, vegetables, legumes, garlic, and almonds. And let's not forget the most quintessentially Spanish food of all: olive oil, the centerpiece of Spain's traditional high-fiber, low-fat Mediterranean diet. Spain is the number one producer of olive oil in the world, responsible for more than a third of the world's supply.

Spanish food tends to be extremely simple—improvisational in nature and built around whatever happens to be growing nearby. Spanish cooking is the product of fresh local ingredients and uncomplicated recipes. The Spanish also benefit from a relatively laid-back lifestyle and an enviably healthy attitude toward food. Any first-time visitor to Spain will notice how the locals linger for hours in tapas bars or spend an entire afternoon picking over Sunday lunch.

WHAT'S IN IT

Garlic: This tiny but pungent allium is an all-purpose ingredient in Spanish cooking—the country's number two ingredient after olive oil. One of the most popular Spanish sauces, aïoli, is a combination of these two ubiquitous ingredients—a blend of crushed garlic and olive oil. The Spanish incorporate garlic into the widest range of recipes imaginable: garlic soup, garlic shrimp, garlic bread, garlic chicken—there's no end of delicious recipes featuring this ingredient. You really can't go wrong with garlic: it has an antibacterial property that prevents infections and destroys health-harmful blood clots, and it can lower your blood pressure and reduce the risk of heart attack and stroke.

Saffron: Saffron is the single most expensive spice in the world, but a little goes a long way. The Spanish love saffron, which gives their national dish, paella, its characteristic bright yellow color. Saffron, which is sold in threads, adds a delicate flavor to foods. It's also been shown to help fight tumors and reverse the effects of brain damage from drinking alcohol.

Beverage of Choice: Red Wine

Like the French and Italians, the Spanish typically enjoy a glass of red wine with dinner. In Spain, wine is primarily drunk as an accompaniment to a meal—an extension of the joy the Spanish take in dining together.

Almonds: Almonds, which grow all over the Andalusia region of southern Spain, pop up in all sorts of Spanish dishes. Many typical Spanish sweets—including macaroons, marzipan, and nougat—are almond based. In general, I don't recommend nuts as a source of protein because they have a fairly high fat content, deriving more than three-fourths of their calories from fat. Almonds, however, with the highest protein content of any nut, are packed with nutrients—manganese, magnesium, vitamin E, and folic acid, among others—and have been shown to lower the risk of heart disease. Almonds also contain vitamin B_{17}, or laetrile, which has been shown to fight cancer. As a garnish, almonds can be a healthy alternative to butter, but it's important to remember that they're roughly 80 percent fat.

Citrus Fruits: Beautiful citrus fruits—oranges, blood oranges, and clementines—flourish in southern Spain. The Spanish regularly cook with citrus fruits; they garnish lobster with oranges and toss clementines on top of salads. For dessert, they might serve blood oranges soaked in red wine. Another popular fruit native to Spain is the pomegranate, a mainstay of the Spanish diet for its antioxidant properties.

Beans and Legumes: No Spanish pantry is complete without a wide selection of dried beans, which are inexpensive and provide a fat-free, nutrient-dense source of vegetable protein. Beans come in dozens of varieties, and the Spanish never get bored with them.

Garbanzos (the Spanish name for chickpeas) are popular all over the Mediterranean region, from the Middle East to Italy. They're a great source of fiber that can help decrease cholesterol. Garbanzos also can prevent blood sugar levels from rising too fast after a meal, stalling the release of insulin and stabilizing metabolic processes.

Cooking Oil of Choice: Olive

Like other cultures in the Mediterranean region, the Spanish use olive oil on absolutely everything and at every stage of a meal. They use it for cooking, seasoning, and even dipping. So they should be bursting out of their pants, right? Not so.

Olive oil, the main source of fat in the Mediterranean diet, is actually one of the healthiest foods you can eat. Research has shown that people who regularly consume olive oil have a lower risk of heart disease, breast cancer, osteoporosis, and rheumatoid arthritis.

That's because olive oil—which the Spanish call "liquid gold"—is high in monounsaturated fat, which raises your "good" (HDL) cholesterol while lowering your artery-clogging "bad" (LDL) cholesterol. Olive oil also contains anti-inflammatory antioxidants that can protect your arteries, which is one big reason the Spanish have such a low incidence of heart disease. And it's a source of polyphenols, flavonoids, and vitamin E.

Lima beans and fava beans (Asturian *fabes*) also make frequent appearances on the Spanish table. Lentil stew is a standard dish in Spain, and restaurant meals often start with a small plate of filling *lentejas*.

Seafood: Since so much of the Iberian Peninsula touches the water, it's only logical that seafood features prominently in the Spanish diet. In Spain's world-famous fish markets, you can buy all sorts of fish. Trout, shrimp, crabs, squid, mussels, and lobsters are often cooked in lemon juice and a little olive oil, then served in a simple tomato- or garlic-based sauce.

Ham: Wild Iberian pigs, which eat a diet of acorns, produce what many consider to be the finest ham in the world: *jamón ibérico,* though seldom a main course, spices up a great variety of foods. Chorizo—salted, cured pork—adds a kick to many dishes. Although both are great additions to soups and main dishes, be sure to use them sparingly, as they are very high in saturated fat.

Seviche: Cooking Without Heat

Seviche is one of my all-time favorite Latin American dishes, and you don't even need a stove to prepare it (unless you're making shellfish seviche, which is usually cooked). *Seviche* refers to any fish marinated in a mixture of citrus juices, usually lemon and lime, though occasionally orange and grapefruit as well. The citric acid has a pickling effect on the fish, effectively cooking it without heat. Although seviche originated in Peru, it has become a mainstay of diets all over Latin America and Spain. Ecuadorans eat seviche with tomato sauce, Costa Ricans with minced onions and cilantro, Chileans with garlic and red peppers, and Peruvians with corn. However it is served, seviche is hands down one of the healthiest foods on the planet.

HOW THEY PREPARE IT

Stewing: Every region in Spain has its own type of stew, and the Spanish language has at least half a dozen words for this dish. Hearty, one-dish meals of vegetables and meat are typical of Spain's cuisine.

Sautéing: Lightly sautéing shrimp and other fish in olive oil is a common cooking technique in Spain.

Roasting: Roasting is a popular way to prepare meat in Spanish cuisine.

HOW THEY EAT IT

They keep their meals simple—and local.

Simplicity is the cornerstone of the best Spanish cuisine. Spain has a big rural population and strong agricultural traditions, and the Spanish still favor foods grown in their own regions—or even their own backyards. People who live in coastal areas such as Galicia eat a lot of seafood. Inhabitants of mountainous regions such as Catalonia and the Basque Country seldom go a day without eating the mushrooms that grow wild in the Pyrenees. In the sun-drenched south, tomatoes are part of almost

---

The Snack That's a Meal: Tapas

Nothing typifies the Spanish fondness for leisurely nibbling like tapas, Spain's answer to Greece's mezes, Italy's antipasti, and South Korea's banchan.

The word *tapa* means "lid," a reference to the saucer that waiters would place over wineglasses to ward off the flies in the days before air-conditioning. Over time, they began adding almonds, anchovies, or olives—whatever food was handy at the moment—to these little saucers, and the tradition of tapas was born.

To this day, tapas are a bar food. The Spanish often enjoy them standing up, while leaning against the counter chatting with friends. They might order one dish or ten, depending on how hungry they are or how much time they have on their hands. Eating tapas is a social affair, an excuse to keep the conversation going—the very opposite of an all-you-can-eat buffet.

Examples of classic tapas include *tortilla española* (an egg omelet often made with leftover fried potatoes); *patatas bravas* (potato chunks fried in olive oil); cured ham and native manchego cheese; *chorizo al vino* (Spanish sausage cooked in wine); and *gambas al ajillo* (shrimp sautéed in garlic and olive oil).

Although tapas have gotten more elaborate in recent years, the basic principle is unchanged: they are small dishes to be consumed slowly, in the company of friends. Other than that, there are no rules about how to mix and match various tapas. As in so much Spanish food, it's all about personal taste and experimentation.

---

every meal. Gazpacho was invented in Andalusia, the southernmost part of Spain that almost touches Africa.

They make pleasure a priority.

Yes, I know, this advice sounds obvious to the point of idiocy, but it does bear repeating, especially in countries such as Spain that have taken the "live to eat" ethos to new heights.

The Spanish take great pride in their native culinary traditions, and they love, love, *love* to eat. In Spain, dinner isn't just about the food on your plate. It's a supremely social affair, an excuse to kick back for hours and hours with your friends and family. It's no coincidence that the Spanish national dish, paella, is traditionally eaten straight from the pan, with friends and family gathered around one big dish. The first time I ate paella, in Barcelona, I couldn't believe that a single-dish meal could explode with so many different colors and flavors. I was so full afterward that dessert was not even an option.

They improvise freely.

Anything goes—that's the key lesson of tapas and Spanish cooking in general. If you're missing an "essential" ingredient, there's no reason to scrap the whole recipe. Play around with whatever you find in your pantry or fridge. Use your imagination to make it work. Tapas, gazpacho, paella—so many Spanish foods are mere templates that can be embellished in a thousand different ways.

HOW THEY BURN IT

Frequent relaxation plays a big role in the healthy Spanish lifestyle. After lunch on weekdays, the Spanish typically lie down for a siesta lasting an hour or even longer. Stores close, businesses put a sign in the front window, and the whole nation shuts down for the hottest hours of the afternoon. Good luck buying aspirin at 2:00 P.M. on a Tuesday!

But did you know that napping—or at least getting eight hours of shut-eye every night—could have major health benefits? Napping regularly can lower your blood pressure and stress levels while increasing on-the-job productivity. Adequate sleep is a crucial part of regulating your metabolism, which is essential for keeping your weight low. A study published in the *International Journal of Obesity* found a correlation between fewer hours of sleep and rising childhood obesity rates.[1] And these days, we're sleeping less than ever. Eighty years ago, adults averaged 8.77 hours of sleep a night. Today, that average has fallen to 6.85 hours.

I'm not saying that a midday snooze is realistic for most nine-to-fivers—of course not! Even in Spain, the realities of modern life have eroded the country's proud tradition of napping. Historically, Spanish government employees worked from 9:00 A.M. to 7:00 or 8:00 P.M., a timetable that factored in an extremely long lunch break. But now the Spanish workday is much more similar to ours, with only one hour off for lunch.

Perhaps an even more important element of Spanish people's overall health is their habit of walking everywhere. Spanish cities are much more compact than ours, designed and constructed long before the invention of the interstate highway and the minivan, so it's easy to get everything you need for day-to-day life within a few blocks of your home. As a result, especially in smaller cities, the Spanish take care of all their daily business on foot. They walk to work, to church, to the doctor, to the tailor. Like the French, they make trips on foot to the grocery store just about every day of the week, usually buying only what they need for the next meal.

In the United States, urbanites who occasionally trade their car keys for a pair of comfortable sneakers also tend to weigh less. A Rutgers University study of 200,000 Americans found that city dwellers weighed on average six pounds less than their suburban counterparts, mostly because they frequently went places on foot.[2]

In Spain, walking is part of the culture. Years ago, the Spanish even formalized a ritual known as the paseo, a Sunday evening stroll that the whole family goes on together. What better way to digest a gigantic Sunday lunch than with a leisurely stroll through town, spent chatting with your family and friends?

DAILY MENU

Breakfast: Breakfast in Spain is a fairly simple affair, consisting of some bread product—toast, a sweet roll, or torrijas (Spanish bread pudding)—with coffee and freshly squeezed orange juice.

Lunch: The Spanish usually eat lunch between 1:30 and 4:00 P.M. As in France, this is typically the largest meal of the day. It might include a light salad or soup (maybe the vegetable-packed gazpacho), lentils with chorizo or another small side dish; then fish, meat, or poultry for the main course.

Dinner: Dinner usually begins around 9:00 P.M. The last meal of the day tends to be light—a salad and some tapas. On special occasions, the family might gather for paella, a wonderful one-dish meal that's a mixture of saffron rice, vegetables, and your choice of protein.

TO-GO TIPS

- Focus on local foods and flavors, building your diet around foods cultivated in your area.
- Don't forget that sometimes the simplest food is also the tastiest.
- Learn to improvise in the kitchen and at the table. Cooking, like eating, should be a creative act, not a form of punishment.
- Indulge—but in moderation.
- Take it easy. Get plenty of rest and carve out time in your day to run errands on foot.

TEN

South Korea

AVERAGE LIFE EXPECTANCY TOTAL POPULATION: 78.72 years

PERCENTAGE OF OVERWEIGHT ADULTS: 43.8 male; 40.2 female

PERCENTAGE OF OBESE ADULTS: 10.1 male; 4.1 female

MEAT CONSUMPTION PER PERSON (2002): 48.0 kg

DIET COMPOSITION (PERCENTAGE OF TOTAL NUTRIENTS):
CARBOHYDRATES: 64
PROTEIN: 13
FAT: 23

Although South Korea's culinary traditions overlap those of China and Japan to a large extent, this country does have its own distinctive cuisine, which is responsible for a very healthy population. The life span of Koreans continues to rise, most recently to 79.1 years. (Note: In this chapter, I'm talking about South Koreans throughout even where "South" is not specified.)

WHAT THEY EAT

Korean food bears a definite resemblance to Chinese and Japanese food. As in many Asian countries, the diet in Korea is built around starches such as rice and noodles, which accompany almost every meal. Soybean derivatives, particularly tofu, are also common. In general, though, the Koreans use less oil than the Chinese, and Korean food tends to be more heavily seasoned—especially so as you move south on the peninsula. Although the Koreans share many dishes with the Japanese—especially fish-based ones such as sashimi—and even the hibachi-style tabletop grill, Japanese food is much blander.

Like many Asians, Koreans consume very few dairy products. Butter is a rare ingredient, used only in special-occasion baked goods. You would never see butter on the dinner table in Korea. Cheese also is rare, an expensive luxury imported from abroad.

WHAT'S IN IT

Kimchi: Kimchi is the most ubiquitous food in Korea. Koreans eat this pickled vegetable dish at just about every meal, so it makes sense that they would have more than two hundred varieties. Koreans have been pickling vegetables for more than a thousand years so that the harvest will last through the long Korean winter. The traditional method of making kimchi involves placing pickled vegetables in pots and burying them in the ground to ferment.

Kimchi is often made from cabbage, but ingredients might also include green onions, radishes, powdered red chiles, garlic, even watermelon rind. It is a nutritional powerhouse, strengthening the immune system, fighting cancer, lowering cholesterol, and even slowing the aging process.[1] Kimchi contains fiber and lactobacillus, a "good" bacteria that speeds digestion and may even fight cancer. When eaten regularly, these two elements can give you a sense of fullness before you even begin a meal.

Cabbage: Cabbage is a good source of fiber, as well as vitamins A, B, C, and E. It contains very little sugar and is very low in calories. Koreans eat cabbage in many different ways; most kimchi is made from this cold-weather, all-terrain vegetable.

Beverage of Choice: Tea

The people of Korea are prodigious tea drinkers. Since ginseng root is native to their land, Koreans have consumed large quantities of ginseng tea for centuries. The name of another traditional Korean tea, *omijacha*, means "five flavors." These flavors are sweet, sour, bitter, salty, and spicy. *Saenggangcha*, or ginger tea, is a Korean tea served hot and enjoyed at cafés, while naturally caffeine-free barley tea is considered a good treatment for a cold. In Korea, as in so many other parts of Asia, there is a tea for every occasion.

Beef: Korean barbecue, prepared on tabletop charcoal grills, is popular throughout the country, although Koreans consume a great deal less beef than we do. The average American eats sixty-seven pounds of beef a year, compared to the sixteen pounds that Koreans eat.[2]

Garlic: Koreans eat exponentially more garlic than the residents of neighboring Asian countries. In fact, the Japanese have a pejorative term for the Koreans: the garlic eaters. Garlic has powerful nutritional properties: it can prevent cancer, fight heart disease, and thin the blood, which results in lower blood pressure. Green onions and hot peppers are often combined with garlic to produce Korea's distinctively spicy sauces.

Lettuce: Koreans wrap their beef dishes not in bread but in lettuce leaves. Korean sashimi (which tends to be larger and chunkier than the Japanese variety) is also typically served inside lettuce leaves.

Ginseng: Ginseng root, which is grown all over Korea, is believed to have medicinal properties. In Korea, ginseng is served as a tea, with honey, or incorporated into other dishes. There is even ginseng wine.

Mushrooms: In Korea, mushrooms are typically served as banchan (tapas) or on top of stir-fried dishes such as *bibimbap*. Mushrooms, which consist of 80 to 90 percent water, are an extremely low-calorie food. They provide potassium, which can lower blood pressure and reduce the risk of a stroke, and selenium, which can protect cells from free radicals in the environment. Shiitake mushrooms have even been used to fight cold and flu symptoms.

> **Cooking Oil of Choice: Sesame or Canola**
>
> Koreans use very little oil, which makes their diet naturally low in fat. When they do use it, like cooks in other Asian countries, they prefer sesame oil or canola oil.

HOW THEY PREPARE IT

Fried foods are virtually unheard of in Korea. Koreans also do very little baking, since the traditional Korean kitchen stove is wood-fired and has no oven. Most Korean foods are made by boiling, blanching, braising, steaming, sautéing, stir-frying, or grilling. Barbecuing is a common method of preparing meat in Korea.

HOW THEY EAT IT

They balance their meals.

The "five flavors" approach to cooking, *omijacha* (see box page 82), is another trait that Korea shares with Chinese and Japanese cuisine. The most famous Korean dish, *bibimbap,* is an illustration of this ancient principle, with ingredients that correspond to the five elements in nature: wood, fire, earth, metal, and water and stimulate all five senses. *Bibimbap,* which means "stirred rice" or "stirred meal," is a mixture of fried rice, meat, and seasoned vegetables, usually topped with a fried egg and chile pepper paste. *Bibimbap* also represents the principle of yin and yang, or the balance of all opposing forces in the universe. This philosophical approach to food is evident in many aspects of Korean cuisine.

HOW THEY BURN IT

Many traditional martial arts, including tae kwon do and hapkido, originated in Korea, and Koreans of all ages practice these arts of "coordinated grace." Koreans also burn calories as part of their everyday life. Because many Koreans live in urban areas, they tend to much of their daily business on foot.

The Snack That's a Meal: Banchan

Walk into any Korean restaurant, and a platter of complimentary banchan will greet you at the table. Banchan—a series of small, varied dishes—are a traditional meal starter in Korea, similar to tapas, dim sum, or mezes elsewhere in the world. Typical banchan might include small cubes of beef, noodles, pancakes, and of course kimchi. Less expensive restaurants might serve simpler fare, such as bean sprouts or pickled winter vegetables.

DAILY MENU

Breakfast: Breakfast in Korea doesn't differ substantially from other meals; it's just smaller. A typical breakfast includes rice, soup, and seasoned vegetables. Western-style breakfasts have become more common in recent years, however.

Lunch: For lunch, Koreans might have boiled noodles, anchovies, and sliced zucchini in a broth. Another option would be savory pancakes peppered with scallions and dipped in a mixture of soy sauce, vinegar, and powdered red chiles.

Dinner: Dinner is the main meal of the day in Korea and tends to be a more elaborate version of breakfast and lunch. A typical dinner might feature a pot of boiling stock, like a fondue pot. Using chopsticks, you dip meat and vegetables into the broth to cook them.

TO-GO TIPS

- Make the most of Mother Nature. If you live in a cold climate, learn to love winter vegetables, or learn techniques for preserving your favorite summer produce.
- Enjoy beef—just not too much of it.
- To keep your diet both interesting and healthy, get a good balance of flavors in every meal.
- Add garlic. Garlic makes everything taste better, and it's healthy.

ELEVEN

Israel

AVERAGE LIFE EXPECTANCY TOTAL POPULATION: 80.73 years

PERCENTAGE OF OVERWEIGHT ADULTS: 57.5 male; 57.2 female

PERCENTAGE OF OBESE ADULTS: 24.3 male; 16.2 female

MEAT CONSUMPTION PER PERSON (2002): unavailable

DIET COMPOSITION (PERCENTAGE OF TOTAL NUTRIENTS):
  CARBOHYDRATES: 52
  PROTEIN: 15
  FAT: 33

Israel lies at the center of the Middle East, the region where Europe, Africa, and Asia come together. Successive conquests and control by different empires have shaped the civilizations and cultures of the region, and the diversity of Middle Eastern cuisine reflects this history. The geography of the Middle East also plays a key role in its unique culinary traditions. With coasts, mountains, and deserts all concentrated in a small area, the Middle East produces a huge range of fresh fruits, vegetables, and grains, providing the basis for an extremely varied diet.

I've targeted Israel here because its cuisine reflects many of the best cross-cultural qualities of Middle Eastern cooking, with a few more thrown in for good measure. Even better, Israel is number thirteen on the CIA *World Factbook*'s life expectancy list, with an impressive average life expectancy of 80.73 years.

WHAT THEY EAT

It's no surprise that Israel should have such a remarkably diverse cuisine, since people from so many corners of the earth have settled in the tiny country over the past sixty years. Israeli food is a delicious hybrid of Middle Eastern styles, with contributions from Europe, Russia, North Africa, and even central Asia thrown in. Increasingly and unfortunately, American imports such as pizza and burgers have also made their mark.

Israelis eat many different small salads and dips made from chiles, chickpeas, and garlic. They pair dips such as hummus and baba ghanoush with paper-thin pita bread, the flatbread eaten all over the Middle East. Falafel, or deep-fried balls of ground chickpeas, is another familiar main dish. Various grilled meats and lentil-based soups also play a big part in the country's day-to-day diet. There really is no end to the variety of Israeli fare, which ranges from Iraqi pickled vegetables to Hungarian goulash.

WHAT'S IN IT

Among the most popular ingredients in Israeli cooking are tomatoes, peppers, onions, garlic, lemons, olive oil, dill, and parsley. These are used in all sorts of dishes, including those made with the following items.

Meat: Chicken is the meat of choice in Israel and the Middle East in general. Poorer families have traditionally used bones of other animals to flavor their soups and stews, since they cannot afford the meat itself. This trick makes for an inadvertently healthy way to get the flavor of meat without much of the fat.

Eggplant: This high-fiber, nutrient-rich vegetable has a meaty taste and texture and is high in potassium, manganese, vitamin B_1, and chlorogenic acid (which might have anticancer, antiviral, and antimicrobial properties). Eating eggplant frequently can also lower cholesterol and improve cardiovascular health. In Israel, people eat eggplant grilled, stewed, fried, puréed into a dip (as in baba ghanoush), and pickled.

Turmeric: The bright yellow spice commonly used in curry dishes, turmeric has anti-inflammatory properties that can help cure ailments large and small, from healing cuts to improving cardiovascular health. Scientists are also studying the potential benefits of turmeric in treating Alzheimer's disease, cancer, liver disorders, and depression.[1] As if all that wasn't enough, turmeric has also been shown to fight inflammatory bowel diseases such as Crohn's disease and ulcerative colitis.

Mint: Mint, the most common herb in Middle Eastern cooking, is a great source of manganese and vitamins A and C. It is also used to soothe the stomach and relieve digestive distress. The phytonutrients in mint leaves might protect against cancer, asthma, and allergies.

Chickpeas, Lentils, and Fava Beans: In the Middle East, protein-rich legumes are eaten almost daily. A source of folate, manganese, and fiber, chickpeas can aid in regulating blood sugar and lowering cholesterol. Fava beans, which have similar nutritional properties, are eaten daily by a majority of the population. Lentils are another versatile staple.

Sesame Seeds: Sesame seeds are a nutritional powerhouse—high in manganese, copper, calcium, magnesium, iron, phosphorus, vitamin B_1, zinc, folic acid, protein, and linoleic acid (an unsaturated omega-6 fatty acid)—and Israelis eat them almost every day. Tahini, a peanut-butterlike paste of ground sesame seeds, is a key ingredient in hummus, which is arguably the most versatile food in the Middle East. Sesame seeds can also help lower cholesterol and prevent high blood pressure.

Raisins, Apricots, and Pomegranates: Middle Easterners frequently finish their meals with these antioxidant-rich fruits, which are used in all sorts of preparations.

Pita Bread: Pita, a type of leavened flatbread, is often eaten with every meal of the day. If you compare a pita pocket to a slice of white bread or a bagel, it's hard to see any similarities between the two foods. The

Beverage of Choice: Coffee with Cardamom

The Israelis drink lots of coffee, with cardamom added for an extra twist. Cardamom, an herb in the ginger family, is also a popular flavoring in Indian food. Indians use cardamom in traditional ayurvedic medicine as a digestive stimulant.

density is so different: pita is thin and hollow, with a fraction of the calories of even one slice of white bread and less than half the calories of a bagel (and twice the fiber).

Bulgur: Bulgur, a type of cracked wheat, is the basis of the popular Middle Eastern salad tabouli. Bulgur is a whole grain and high in fiber, which can lower the risk of certain cancers. Bulgur is also low in fat and very filling.

Yogurt: Lactobacillus and other "good" bacteria in yogurt are extremely beneficial to the digestive system. The high calcium content of yogurt helps build strong, healthy bones. In the Middle East, yogurt is often eaten unsweetened, in its pure form.

Greek, or strained, yogurt, called *labneh* in Israel, requires twice as much milk to make as traditional yogurt, but it has significantly more protein and less sugar, and it is much thicker (and more delicious).

HOW THEY PREPARE IT

With the obvious exception of falafel, very few dishes are fried in Israel. Most are grilled (think kebabs) or baked. Meat dishes are prepared with great simplicity, often grilled with a mixture of spices, with no fatty sauces added.

HOW THEY EAT IT

They cook at home.

Although vendors of street food such as vegetarian falafel and meat kebabs have always been a mainstay of life in Israel and the entire

> ### Cooking Oil of Choice: Vegetable
>
> Coastal areas of the Middle East cook with olive oil, while wealthier segments of the population use ghee, or clarified butter. In recent years, however, cheap vegetable oils (more than olive oil) have become the most common cooking base—to the detriment of the population's health.

Middle East, until the twentieth century, sit-down restaurants were virtually unheard of. Even today, many families eat at home the vast majority of the time.

They mix it up.

As I've already said, a wide range of nationalities and cultures are represented on just about every street and in every kitchen in Israel. Walk through any neighborhood, and you will encounter foods from Europe, the Balkans, North Africa, and the Arab Middle East. Israeli cuisine is a combination of these and other diverse influences.

HOW THEY BURN IT

Because Israelis are required to join the army at the age of eighteen, they establish a strong foundation of fitness early in their adolescence. They also return to basic training for one month every year through middle age.

DAILY MENU

Breakfast: Unlike in the West, where different types of food are eaten at different times of the day (eggs or cereal for breakfast, sandwich for lunch, steak for dinner), people in Israel eat the same foods in different forms around the clock. Breakfast usually consists of leftovers from other meals. One example is whole wheat pita bread dipped in *labneh* (a thick, strained Greek-style yogurt), olive oil, or za'atar (a traditional Middle Eastern blend of spices). An Israeli might also start the day with hard-boiled eggs, slow-cooked fava beans, olives, or falafel. My all-time favorite Israeli breakfast is *shakshuka,* a dish of scrambled eggs stewed with tomatoes, garlic, onions, and spices. Delicious!

Lunch: In Israel, the largest meal of the day traditionally is lunch. A typical lunch might consist of a lamb stew made with onions, tomato paste, and eggplant, or shish kebabs (grilled meat served on skewers). Kebabs are typically a street or restaurant food, eaten on the go rather than in the home. Israelis also might have a falafel sandwich for lunch, or a pita stuffed with eggplant, hard-boiled eggs, and tahini.

Dinner: Historically, Middle Easterners ate only a light snack in the evening, but as the region has become more prosperous (and Westernized), more and more people have adopted our three-meal-a-day routine. A dinner might include stuffed eggplant and a chicken salad, with sides of rice, bulgur, or pita bread. In Israel, a soup followed by some form of grilled meat is common at the evening meal.

TO-GO TIPS

- Synthesize the best of what the world has to offer every time you sit down to eat. The diversity of the Israeli diet is a big part of what keeps Israelis so healthy.
- Try eating your sandwiches on thinner bread, such as pita. That way, you will get all the flavor and convenience of bread without all the calories.
- Go skinny-dipping! By learning to make your own vegetable dips, you can squeeze good nutrients into the busiest schedule.
- Eat at home more often. You will have more control over the content and size of your meals.

TWELVE

Greece

AVERAGE LIFE EXPECTANCY TOTAL POPULATION: 79.66 years

PERCENTAGE OF OVERWEIGHT ADULTS: 61.3 male; 75.7 female

PERCENTAGE OF OBESE ADULTS: 24.5 male; 27.7 female

MEAT CONSUMPTION PER PERSON (2002): 78.7 kg

DIET COMPOSITION (PERCENTAGE OF TOTAL NUTRIENTS):
    CARBOHYDRATES: 53
    PROTEIN: 13
    FAT: 34

I couldn't leave Greece and the world famous Mediterranean diet off my list of finalists—even though Greeks aren't as slim as they used to be. Coming in at number twenty-six on the life expectancy list, Greeks are generally not as healthy as they used to be either, so we will be looking at the *traditional* Greek diet, not its contemporary, fast-food degradation.

In its purest form, the Greek diet typifies what has come to be celebrated as the Mediterranean diet, which has been linked to a lower risk of cancer deaths. A study at the University of Crete found that pregnant women who

---

Beverage of Choice: Coffee

In Greece, as in so many countries throughout Europe, coffee is the favorite beverage. The Greeks like their coffee two ways: "frappé" style, which is made from instant coffee, iced and covered with frothy milk, unfiltered. The Greeks' traditional thick, strong unfiltered coffee has sediment on the bottom and is similar to what we would call Turkish coffee. Both styles are often served sweetened.

---

followed the diet gave birth to children with a lower incidence of allergies and asthma. And over the long term, the Mediterranean diet can reduce the risk of diabetes, lower blood pressure, and decrease "bad" cholesterol.

WHAT THEY EAT

The traditional Greek diet is built around olive oil, fresh local vegetables, whole grains, legumes, and fish high in omega-3 fatty acids, with only a little meat thrown in on occasion. People who eat this way have remarkably low levels of heart disease and even lower obesity rates. Although the contemporary Greek diet has deviated from this ideal, with refined grains, high-fat cheeses, and fast foods occupying an ever more prominent place on the menu, the basic principles behind the original Mediterranean diet are worthy of our attention.

WHAT'S IN IT

In addition to the following foods, Greeks eat a lot of tomatoes, eggplant, onions, green beans, and green peppers. These and other vegetables make up a large part of every meal. Nuts and seeds are also important components of the traditional Greek diet.

Fresh Seafood: Greece is a peninsula surrounded by several islands, so it makes sense that the people would eat heart-healthy fish on a daily basis. Just about any fish you can name—halibut, red mullet, swordfish, tuna, sardines, whitefish, and shrimp—is part of Greek cuisine. Oily fish such as sardines are good sources of protein and omega-3s.

Cooking Oil of Choice: Olive

Although the average Greek derives up to 40 percent of his or her daily calories from fat, Greeks still have one of the healthiest diets in the world. That's because they get most of their fat from olive oil, a monounsaturated fat that lowers "bad" (LDL) cholesterol without reducing "good" (HDL) cholesterol. Olive oil is high in calories, but it remains in the stomach longer than carbs or protein and stimulates hormones, which can suppress your appetite and create a feeling of fullness. One study found that a Mediterranean diet containing olive oil was more effective at long-term weight loss than a low-fat diet.[1] After eighteen months, only 20 percent of the women on the low-fat diet had stuck to their eating regime. By contrast, the women on the Mediterranean diet said that they didn't feel as if they were dieting at all.

Leafy Greens: The traditional Greek diet has leafy dark green vegetables in plentiful supply. Leafy greens contain lutein and other vitamins and minerals essential for good cardiovascular health. Today, Greeks eat salads regularly.

Kalamata Olives: Kalamata olives, native to Greece, are mainly fat, but they are also an excellent source of vitamin E. Eaten in moderation, they can be great in salads and other dishes.

Legumes: Like other Mediterraneans, Greeks eat a variety of legumes, including chickpeas and lima beans.

Whole Grains: Greeks eat barley and other whole grains in their bread products. Greek breads tend to have a much higher nutritional value than the overly processed white breads that too often dominate Americans' diet.

HOW THEY PREPARE IT

Grilling fresh meat and fish is the most common way to prepare food in Greece.

> ### The Snack That's a Meal: Mezes
>
> Greeks have a long tradition of eating mezes, a series of small dishes designed to be picked at slowly over the course of a long evening. Typical Greek mezes include stuffed grape leaves, tzatziki (yogurt with cucumbers), fava bean purée, and grilled meat.

HOW THEY EAT IT

The Greeks eat family style, gathered around the table and sharing large dishes. Eating at home is a critical element of this tradition. Today, however, more than one in ten Greek teenagers eat unhealthy fast food at least five times a week.[2]

HOW THEY BURN IT

The gymnasium and the Olympic Games were both inventions of the ancient Greeks, but today Greeks get less and less exercise. Maybe that's one reason 68.5 percent of them are overweight! In the past, the typical Greek villager would conduct all his or her daily business on foot, walking to the store, the office, the doctor, and so on. Today, more and more Greeks are driving just about everywhere.

DAILY MENU

Breakfast: A typical Greek breakfast usually includes some type of pastry and a cup of strong Greek coffee. Greeks might also eat honey spread on toast. Today, more and more Greek children are leaving home without eating breakfast—a habit that is contributing to the country's rising obesity rate.

Lunch: For lunch, Greeks might have a traditional Greek salad with tomatoes, cucumbers, feta, and olives. A gyro—pork, lamb, or chicken stuffed in a pita along with yogurt sauce and garnishes of tomato and onion—is a popular Greek street food often eaten for lunch. You can easily make a gyro at home with skinless chicken breast or another healthy protein.

Dinner: Dinner might include another fresh salad; some local fish; and several side dishes, perhaps tzatziki and some vegetables, such as green beans and tomatoes.

TO-GO TIPS

- Build your diet around legumes, whole grains, and leafy green vegetables.
- Choose thick, filling Greek-style yogurt (nonfat, of course) for maximum calcium—and maximum satisfaction.
- Don't be afraid of fat—as long as it's the good kind, such as that found in olive oil.
- Try adding small fish to your diet (i.e. herring or sandines), as they are lower in mercury than larger fish. The Greeks know that local fish are a great staple in any diet, adding both protein and healthy fat.

PART 3

THE 5-FACTOR WORLD DIET ACTION PLAN

THIRTEEN

Understanding the 5-Factor Edge

Now that we have the lessons from our Top 10 countries under our belts, so to speak, we can get to the fun part: putting those lessons into practice. In the coming chapters, we're going to combine all these lessons to create one expansive plan—a new way of thinking about eating (and living) that's guaranteed to keep your routine interesting and international. I'll be modifying these recipes slightly to optimize their nutritional profiles, so don't be surprised to see quinoa substituted for couscous in an Israeli recipe, or brown rice instead of white in sushi. Don't expect exact replicas of your favorite international recipes, but do know that I've made these changes in the interests of health—and convenience. But before we get started with what to eat specifically—and how to shop for it and prepare it—it's important that you understand the guiding principles behind my 5-Factor technique.

THE 5-FACTOR EDGE

Although I outlined the basics of 5-Factor eating in the introduction, it's worth going over these principles again here. First, people on my plan eat five times a day, a system that's been scientifically proven to provide the optimal balance for maintaining healthy and stable insulin levels. My 5-Factor meals also tend to be very easy to make, with no more than five major ingredients per recipe.

If you stick to this eating system six days a week, you can take the seventh as a "free day," when you can eat whatever you want, whenever you want (within reason, of course). I'm not suggesting that you follow the 5-Factor framework religiously, but do bear in mind that people in some of the healthiest countries on the planet enjoy the benefits of small, frequent meals. All over the world, people are living the 5-Factor way without even knowing it!

When it comes to the composition of each of those five daily meals, I have (you guessed it!) five basic criteria.

Criterion 1: Protein

Every meal should include a low-fat, high-quality protein, such as chicken breast, fish, shellfish, egg whites, or yogurt. Protein is a crucial part of a healthy diet for several reasons. First, unlike carbohydrates and fat, our bodies cannot store protein, and so we must ingest protein at regular intervals throughout the day. Second, although carbs and dietary fat can easily be converted to body fat, protein is far less likely to be. Third, a steady intake of protein will help you maintain lean tissue and burn fat. Fourth, protein can boost your metabolism. And finally, protein can give you a feeling of satiety, putting a stop to the bottomless cravings that other foods trigger. That's why we need protein in every meal.

But remember, some proteins are healthier than others: Eating a big handful of nuts or a huge chunk of cheddar cheese might make you feel full, but it will also add an excessive amount of calories and fat to your diet. Some examples of healthy proteins from the World Diet countries are salmon teriyaki from Japan, tofu from China, chickpeas from Israel, roast chicken from France, yogurt from Greece, and seviche from Spain.

Criterion 2: Carbohydrates

There's nothing wrong with eating a high-carb diet, but Americans have a tendency to favor less healthy carbs that are either used as an immediate energy source or converted and stored as fat. The 5-Factor World Diet focuses on carbs such as whole grains and vegetables that release energy slowly and take the body more time to digest. Carbohydrates are absolutely essential to any healthy diet, but not all carbs are created equal.

The key difference between healthy and less healthy carbohydrates is fiber, which affects the rate at which the body can absorb and assimilate foods. You need to make more room on your plate for high-fiber carbohydrates that make you feel fuller faster and for longer periods. These carbs will moderate your blood sugar and energy levels, as well as your appetite. Most of the carbs I recommend fall into this category.

Less healthy carbs, such as table sugar and white bread, break down too quickly in the body, triggering a rapid increase in blood sugar, which in turn causes the release of insulin and makes you more prone to convert foods to body fat. Eating less healthy carbs also makes you more likely to experience a precipitous drop in blood sugar soon after eating, a phenomenon that can destabilize your mood and reactivate your hunger soon afterward.

Whole-grain breads, such as those favored in Sweden, are a much healthier alternative to the white breads, bagels, and deep-dish pizzas we scarf down. Legumes, such as the lentils popular in Spain and France or the chickpeas favored in Italy and Israel, are another source of healthy carbohydrates. And don't forget that many fruits and vegetables also qualify as carbohydrates.

Criterion 3: Fiber

Every meal should include 5 to 10 grams of fiber, a requirement that can generally be satisfied by criterion 2 if you choose a fibrous carbohydrate. Fiber is a carbohydrate that the body doesn't store or convert to energy. It is not found in foods from animal sources, such as meat and dairy products, which is yet another reason that Americans' meat-centered diet can cause health problems. Fiber plays an essential role in maintaining healthy digestion. First, fiber can help stabilize blood sugar. Second, it can slow down digestion, which makes you feel full longer. Equally, important, fiber has been shown to reduce the risk of heart disease, diabetes, some cancers, and other serious health problems.

You can get fiber from many different sources. Insoluble fiber, or "roughage," which provides the bulk in bowel movements, is found in whole grains (enriched breads, oats, bulgur, wheat bran), veggies (cabbage, bok choy, kale, broccoli), fruits, and legumes. Soluble fiber, which draws water into your bowels, is present in oats, barley, beans, lentils, peas, nuts, seeds, apples, and other fruits and vegetables. World Diet fiber sources include legumes, whole-grain breads, whole-grain noodles (preferably cooked al dente, because undercooked pasta takes a little longer to digest and will therefore make you feel fuller longer), and whole-grain breakfast cereals. To get more fiber (and much less fat) out of your protein sources, consider substituting legumes (chickpeas, lentils, fava beans) for two-thirds of the meat in chili and soup recipes.

Criterion 4: Healthy Fat

If your meal includes a fat, make sure it's a healthy one, such as olive oil, fish oil, or canola oil. Fats are a necessary part of every diet, but it's important to remember that they're more than twice as calorically dense as carbohydrates or proteins, so you want to eat them sparingly. Eating too much fat can increase your risk of certain cancers, kidney failure, stroke, and heart disease. Saturated fats in particular can increase your "bad" (LDL) cholesterol. By contrast, unsaturated fats can actually improve your cholesterol profile.

There are two types of unsaturated fats, monounsaturated and polyunsaturated. Monounsaturated fat is present in some vegetable oils (canola oil, olive oil), avocados, almonds, cashews, and sesame seeds. Polyunsaturated fat is present in other vegetable oils (corn oil, sunflower oil), walnuts, and foods that contain omega-3 fatty acids (albacore tuna, sardines, salmon, flaxseeds). Omega-3 fatty acids are the healthiest fats you can include in your diet. That's just one reason why eating fish is so important. When consumed in moderation, foods with unsaturated fats give you a feeling of satiety without contributing to heart disease.

In many of my Top 10 countries, people by no means shy away from "bad" fats—the ones found in cheese and meat—but they eat them in moderation and in much smaller quantities than Americans do. And note that with the exception of Sweden, on my lists of favorite foods in chapters 3–12, there's no mention of margarine, commercial baked goods, processed snack foods, and fast foods such as French fries, all of which contain trans fats. You should avoid trans fats at all costs.

Criterion 5: Beverage

The last component of a healthy 5-Factor meal is a low-calorie, sugar-free beverage. Make your beverage count. Drinking at least eight 8-ounce glasses of fluid a day is the standard recommendation—a practice that can help keep your body hydrated, flush out the toxins, and make you feel full. Steer clear of beverages with a high calorie content. Wouldn't you rather save those calories for your food?

5-FACTOR WORLD DIET BEVERAGE SUGGESTIONS

My Top 10 countries offer a range of beverage options that meet my 5-Factor criteria. In France, there's mineral water. All over Asia, there's green tea—a calorie-free drink with a moderate caffeine content and invaluable antioxidant properties. Chinese oolong tea, which can boost your metabolism, is a satisfying pick-me-up on a workday. People in many of my favorite countries, including Sweden, Italy, Israel, and France, drink coffee regularly, but I should point out that coffee in these countries has almost nothing in common with the coffee-flavored sugar bombs that have become so popular in the United States over the past decade.

Tea: Experiment with all sorts of tea, including black, oolong, green, ginseng, and African red bush tea. Serve tea piping hot or over ice—however you like it! Kombucha, a type of fermented tea, is an increasingly popular beverage choice in the United States. Try it! You can find it in the refrigerated beverage section of any health food store.

Water: Flat or sparkling, tap or imported—drink it however you like it best. Try sprucing up your water with a squeeze of lemon, lime, or orange or a slice of cucumber.

Your Weekly Free Day

Your once-weekly free day is as important a part of the 5-Factor World Diet as any of the other guidelines. The Italians do it—why shouldn't you? Eating whatever you want (in moderation, of course) one day a week will prevent you from feeling deprived, which has led to the failure of many a diet. My theory is that eating badly one day a week is a lot better for you in the long run than eating semi-badly seven days a week. And who knows—once you get on the 5-Factor bandwagon, you might find that you no longer crave the same greasy, high-sugar, trans fatty foods that used to rock your world.

Wine is a great example of an occasional free-day indulgence. I'm not encouraging you to drink it on a daily basis, but one glass a week won't hurt you. The moderate consumption of wine does not contribute to obesity, and some studies have shown that red wine in particular can be good for your heart. All that being said, no one's life has ever been shortened by too little wine! Wine contains no essential nutrients or minerals, and it's not exactly low-calorie or filling. In fact, alcohol is nearly twice as calorically dense as carbohydrates and proteins. That's why I suggest that you treat it as a free-day treat, not as an everyday necessity.

Coffee: Coffee is endlessly variable. Drink it hot or cold; make it in a percolator, a French press, or an espresso machine. Espresso comes in many forms—macchiato, cappuccino, latte—simply by adding nonfat milk. Add cardamom to your coffee for an Israeli treat.

Other Options: An occasional diet soda, Fuze Slenderize, or Vitamin Water is permissible as a treat.

Once you master the basic architecture of your new diet, you're halfway home. Now comes the fun part: filling your shopping basket with a new universe of delicious foods!

FOURTEEN

Understanding Ingredients and Planning Your Shopping List

If you commit to the 5-Factor World Diet, you're going to have to get acquainted with parts of your local market that perhaps have been off your radar until now. In this chapter, I provide an aisle-by-aisle shopping list with the most popular ingredients in my Top 10 countries. These are just some suggestions to get you started. It's a good idea to keep these ingredients, or ones like them, in your home for quick and easy meal preparation.

I've organized my list by category, from the very basic foods such as cooking oils that everyone needs to keep on hand to more regionally specific spices and seasonings. Jot down a few appealing items from my list before your next trip to the grocery store. You don't have to load up your cart with all these foods in a single visit, but try to add one or two new items from every category each time you go to the store until you know what you like.

Shopping Savvy

You've probably heard many times that when you're in the supermarket, you should try to stick to the outer aisles as much as possible. That's where all the good stuff is—the fresh produce, dairy products, and meat that you'd find at a typical open-air market in Europe or Asia. Foods lower in nutrients and higher in fats tend to be concentrated in the store's inner aisles. That said, canned and frozen products such as beans and vegetables are not only as nutritionally valuable as their fresh counterparts, but they allow you to prepare a healthy meal for yourself on any given evening without having to shop for fresh ingredients. There can also be a big economic advantage to stocking up on frozen or canned foods. Most of the time, you don't even have to sacrifice flavor to reap these benefits. Some of the best Italian pomodoro sauces are made with canned tomatoes!

MEAT AND FISH

Here's where you can load up on some essential animal proteins—but remember, go light on the red meat. Like the Chinese, you should use red meat as a side dish or even a garnish, not as the main event (except on free days and special occasions, when you can eat whatever you want). Instead, focus on the leaner, healthier meats that the World Diet countries regularly feast on.

Fish: Do you think it's a coincidence that some of the healthiest countries in the world are also the places where people eat fish on a daily basis? Fish is a great dietary staple, as long as you choose the lower-mercury species. Although tuna, mackerel, and swordfish are delicious, they might be contaminated with higher levels of mercury than other fish, so make sure you limit those to two servings a week. There are plenty of fish that you can eat with abandon, however, including tilapia, freshwater trout, anchovies, whitefish, flounder, herring, and skate. Salmon is another great choice. You can also have as much shellfish as you want: lobster, crabs, clams, and shrimp have low mercury levels as well. The following selections from the sea occupy a big part of the daily menu in the World Diet countries, and they all happen to be low in mercury:

- Salmon (Japan)
- Herring (Sweden)
- Shellfish (Spain)
- Mussels (France)
- Whitefish (Greece)

These and other fish are as versatile as they are delicious. As the chefs in the World Diet countries know, it's all in how you season it!

Poultry: Chicken, which the French and Italians eat regularly, is much leaner and healthier than beef—just remember to eat it without the skin. Chicken is a great source of zinc, iron, potassium, and B vitamins. The white meat has half the fat of the dark meat and therefore far fewer calories and more protein per ounce.

Tofu: Do like the Asians and start incorporating some low-fat tofu into your diet. Try it in stir-fries and substitute it for the red meat in pasta dishes. You might grow to love this incredibly versatile food. But buyer beware: although tofu is a vegetable protein, a good deal of the tofu found in grocery stores has the same amount of fat, or even more, than many animal protein options. So when you're shopping for tofu, read the label and look for a product that derives less than 30 percent of its calories from fat. Tofu also comes in different levels of firmness, from supersoft to extra-firm. You might have to run through several taste tests before finding the type you like best. If you're looking for more of a meat substitute, I suggest erring on the side of firmness—go for tofu that has a texture more like cheese and less like Jell-O. The firmer varieties work better in most recipes. If you're having trouble figuring out which brand and type of tofu is right for you, visit Theworlddiet.com for a list of great-tasting possibilities.

PRODUCE

I usually start my shopping here—the most useful section of the store for our purposes. Fruits and vegetables should be the foundation of your diet. Start expanding your repertoire to include items you might never have tried before. Here are my suggestions, from the mundane to the exotic:

Vegetables

Leafy Greens: You can never go wrong with a serving of leafy greens, a category of super-healthy vegetables that includes bok choy and cabbage—among the most popular vegetables in China. The Greeks also eat a good deal of leafy greens, including kale, which provides sky-high levels of folic acid, vitamin C, potassium, magnesium, and a wide range of phytonutrients such as lutein and beta-carotene.

Seaweed: I know it might sound funny, but the Japanese eat seaweed every day; there's no more naturally salty veggie out there. Try a fresh seaweed salad at a Japanese restaurant, and if you like the taste, look for it in dried form in the international aisle of your supermarket. Nori and wakame are the two kinds of seaweed I use most frequently in my recipes. Seaweed is a fantastic "transport mechanism" that can be an everyday substitute for bread. Instead of wrapping your meal in thick slices of white bread, put it inside a thin sheet of seaweed, which is basically pure fiber. In part IV, I have several delicious meal suggestions that showcase seaweed's many uses.

Leeks: The French know that leeks can be as versatile as onions, and they're also incredibly good for you. Other frequently used French vegetables include eggplant and zucchini.

Tomatoes: Tomatoes are familiar to the American palate, but too often we eat them in the form of pasta and pizza sauces. The Italians, Israelis, Greeks, Swedes, and French enjoy fresh, lycopene-packed tomatoes in all sorts of dishes, sometimes more than once a day.

Mushrooms: In Japan, China, Korea, France, and Spain—that's half of the World Diet countries—mushrooms make an appearance at several meals a week. Mushrooms are both filling and extremely low-calorie, and they come in numerous varieties, so you'll never get bored experimenting with them.

Fruits

Keeping fresh fruit in your house is always a good idea—it makes a great dessert or snack. Instead of drinking fruit juice, reach for a piece of fruit, and if possible choose fruits with edible skin or edible seeds for a fiber boost. Citrus is also a good choice. In Italy, Singapore, and Spain, it's customary to have fruit for dessert, and the Swedish frequently end their meals with a bowl of fresh berries. Why not go out on a limb and try a fruit you've never tasted before? Mangosteen, rambutan, figs, apricots, and pomegranates are all popular dessert picks in the World Diet countries.

DAIRY

Dairy products have gotten a bad rap over the past decade, but don't buy into the hype. Rich in protein, calcium, and vitamin D, dairy is hands down one of the most perfect foods for the human body. And though half of my Top 10 countries (especially those in Asia) consume almost no dairy, quite a few others eat yogurt on a daily basis. In France, Sweden, Greece, and Israel, yogurt is an integral part of the diet. Try plain nonfat yogurt with fruit for a satisfying snack. Avoid high-fat and sugar-laden yogurt. If possible, choose Greek yogurt or an Icelandic form of yogurt called skyr. Both are much higher in protein and essentially lactose-free.

COOKING OILS

Olive Oil: All over the Mediterranean, cooks prefer the heart-healthy "liquid gold"—olive oil. Olive oil is a great source of unsaturated fat and an extremely versatile cooking base. Keep it in your kitchen at all times. Fine, you might say, but which type? I hear you: shopping for olive oil can be a daunting experience. There's virgin, extra virgin, and even pure. How are you to choose from so many varieties that look so much alike? I suggest that you pick up virgin olive oil for cooking and the slightly more expensive extra virgin for salad dressings, which allows you to appreciate the oil's subtle flavoring. Both virgin and extra virgin are distilled from the first pressing of the olives and are extremely high quality. Lower-grade oils, which do not carry the virgin label, might be called "pure olive oil" or "refined olive oil." Only if you see "virgin" or "extra virgin" on the label can you be 100 percent sure that you're getting the real thing.

Canola Oil: Used all over Asia, canola oil is another cooking base with a low saturated fat content. With its omega-3 fatty acids, canola oil can be very heart-healthy. Try it in Asian stir-fries and other everyday basics.

Peanut Oil and Sesame Oil: Many Asian recipes for stir-fries call for either peanut or sesame oil to add flavor to the dish. Keep both oils in your kitchen to give your veggies a little more punch.

WHOLE GRAINS

One habit we will *not* be borrowing from the French is their fondness for white baguettes, which have no more dietary value than Wonder bread. But there are quite a few whole-grain breads and other foods that you could consider adding to your diet.

Flatbreads: Be careful not to go overboard in the bread section, but consider trying flatbreads, such as pitas, which are eaten all over the Mediterranean. Try to find whole-grain versions. Chapati, one of the many Indian foods that has become an essential part of the Singaporean diet, is easy to make on your own if you have the time and desire. Just look online for a recipe. The only ingredients you need are whole-grain flour, water, salt, and the cooking oil of your choice.

Whole-Grain Breads: The pumpernickel and rye breads that the Swedes love have a much higher fiber content and provide more lasting energy than the overly processed white breads that we (and, yes, the French) commonly eat. The density of these dark breads also gives you a feeling of satiety that lighter breads do not. I absolutely love dark breads. Feldkamp is one great brand. Mestemacher (available from Whole Foods and Cost Plus) is one of my all-time favorite brands. The company sells six different types of bread—all very dark—in the United States.

Rice: The number one staple of the Asian diet, rice (especially enriched and whole-grain varieties) can be a nourishing source of carbohydrates. With more than two-thirds of the people in the world consuming white rice as their primary energy source, it's hard to condemn the tiny white grain. However, I suggest opting for brown rice, which is higher in fiber and more nutritious. Another great choice is Bhutanese red rice, which is eaten in the Himalayas. (If you have trouble finding it in your local store, check out WorldPantry.com, or visit Theworlddiet.com for more shopping ideas.) Wild rice is a favorite of mine—but did you know that it's not even part of the rice family? Wild rice is actually a vegetable, and an unbelievably delicious one at that. Black rice is another popular form.

Noodles: Noodles are another international favorite, but why not try some healthier alternatives to your traditional spaghetti? Brown rice noodles, udon noodles, whole wheat pasta, shirataki (seaweed noodles), cellophane or glass (mung bean) noodles, and especially soba (buckwheat) noodles— all of which play a major role in the Japanese diet—are great options worth exploring. They tend to be denser and more filling than the noodles Americans usually eat. Shirataki are thin, translucent, gelatinous, Japanese noodles made from the konjak plant. The word *shirataki* means "white waterfall," which is a pretty apt description of these noodles. Largely composed of water and glucomannan, a water-soluble dietary fiber, they are very low in carbohydrates, fat-free, and high in fiber. You can buy both traditional shirataki and tofu shirataki online at LoCarbU.com.

Bulgur: Bulgur, a type of cracked wheat, is eaten in Greece and throughout the Middle East. It is a wonderfully wholesome alternative to more refined grains. If you can't find bulgur in the rice aisle, head to the bulk foods section of your local health food store.

LEGUMES AND BEANS

As the diet of just about every country on my Top 10 list indicates, legumes are an essential part of a healthy diet. Beyond being high in fiber and low in fat, beans are easy to prepare, easy to store, and easy on the pocketbook, too. They are one of the most versatile proteins you can add to your diet. They fill you up, provide just enough healthy fat, and taste absolutely delicious. You might even consider substituting beans for all or two-thirds of the meat in chili and soup recipes. That's a great way to add nutritional content and subtract fat from your diet. Here are some favorite legumes from across the globe:

- Chickpeas (Spain, Italy, Israel, Greece)
- Cannellini (Italy)
- Lentils (France, Israel, Spain)
- Lima beans (Spain, Greece)

- Fava beans (Greece, Israel)
- Soybeans (Japan)
- Black beans (China)

You can buy most of these legumes either dried or canned in most grocery stores. If you have the time to soak and cook the beans yourself, by all means buy them dried, but if not, don't fret. Canned legumes are often the best bet if you cook in a hurry, and you're not sacrificing any of the food's nutritional properties by taking this shortcut. Fresh legumes are obviously great from a flavor perspective, but canned or frozen beans are also delicious, and preparing your meals with them can be an invaluable time-saver.

SAUCES, SEASONINGS, AND SPICES

With the right mix of seasonings, you can easily add flavor to any dish without adding too many extra calories.

Sauces and Seasonings

Soy Sauce: In China, Korea, Japan, and Singapore, people understand the versatility of soy sauce—which is why they add it to practically every food they eat. Soy sauce is more or less zero-calorie, and it can add zest to soups, stir-fries, and proteins. You should be able to find the low-sodium version at all but the smallest grocery stores.

Other Chinese Sauces: Hoisin sauce and oyster sauce are among the many other Chinese sauces you can use to add zest to your meals. Black bean sauce, another soybean derivative, is great in stir-fries. Look for these sauces in Asian markets or larger grocery stores. Make sure the ones you choose aren't loaded with sugar and artificial ingredients.

Balsamic Vinegar: Balsamic vinegar is one of my all-time favorite foods—an essential ingredient in many salad dressings but also a wonderful addition to a braising liquid. You can even pour it over cut-up fruit for dessert. Balsamic vinegar makes foods taste unbelievably tasty without adding to your calorie load.

Fresh Tomato Sauce: The Italians know that fresh homemade tomato sauce isn't just for pasta. Try using it for squash and other vegetables to create a nutritious side dish.

Spices

Go crazy expanding your spice rack! Experimenting with exotic spices is a great way to give new life to familiar foods—and to boost their health benefits. As with other aspects of this diet, you might already use some of these spices every day in your kitchen; others might be completely unknown to you. Many have anti-inflammatory, antibacterial, and antimicrobial properties. All are worth taking for a spin. Here are a few suggestions, just in case you don't already have them.

Turmeric: This wonder-working spice is used all over Singapore, Japan, and Israel. It has been shown to fight all sorts of diseases, and it adds a striking color to foods.

Saffron: Saffron is expensive, but the Spanish consider this bright yellow spice well worth the investment.

Mint: Middle Easterners use mint on a plethora of foods, and so should you! Add hot water, and you have the most delicious tea in the world.

Herbes de Provence: We use many herbs regularly, but the French *herbes de provence,* a blend of herbs such as rosemary, tarragon, marjoram, sage, and thyme, can't be beat.

Oregano and Basil: These two Italian staples can fight germs and maybe even disease, too—and they taste delicious.

Chili: In Singapore, Japan, China, and Korea, cooks use chili oil and paste, as well as powdered red chiles, in all sorts of dishes. Spicing up your food is a great way to add flavor without fat to just about any meal.

OTHER PANTRY ITEMS

Garlic: Life without garlic would be unthinkable for people in many countries, including Italy, Spain, Korea, and France. You're probably already familiar with the telltale taste (and smell) of this little allium, but

---

DIY Seasoning

To boost taste (and save some money in the process), try growing your own mini-herb garden. You don't even need a yard, just a windowsill that's exposed to regular sunlight. Herbs such as mint, sage, and basil require minimal upkeep, and you never have to worry about running out before making your next recipe.

---

did you know that garlic can lower your blood pressure and reduce your risk of heart attack and stroke? You can buy fresh garlic cloves or use minced canned garlic. I even use dried garlic powder from time to time.

Broth: Broth-based soups are hugely popular everywhere from Japan to France. Chinese and Singaporean diners often start their meals with a light, broth-based soup, which is filling without adding too many calories. As with so many other foods we'll be using, you can choose whether to make your broth from scratch or buy it in either canned or bouillon form. (Whenever possible, choose low-sodium varieties.) In an ideal world, we would make everything ourselves, but many of us (myself included) just don't have the time. The important thing is that you start incorporating these healthy foods into your diet. Don't settle for junk food just because you don't have time to make your own broth.

Tea: I love tea, and so do people throughout the world. Stock your pantry with a variety of teas. Depending on your caffeine preference, you can choose from black tea (higher caffeine content), green tea (moderate caffeine content), oolong tea (similar but slightly higher than green), and decaffeinated herbals. There's no reason to drink calorie-laden sugary sodas when all-natural tea has no calories and tastes delicious.

Coffee: Whether it's instant, espresso, drip, or other, coffee can be a great way to jump-start your energy and temporarily curb your appetite.

Now that you have an overview of the basic ingredients you should be looking for in your local markets, let's turn our attention to how best to prepare all these goodies.

FIFTEEN

Getting Familiar with 5-Factor Cooking Techniques and Tools

It might seem obvious, but it's still worth pointing out that *how* you cook is often as important as *what* you cook. So put aside that deep fryer for a moment and consider some healthier ways to prepare your meal—techniques that people all over the planet have been using for centuries to stay healthy. I've rounded up the ones that are commonly used in my Top 10 countries and (coincidence? I think not) also happen to be extremely healthy. If you haven't yet mastered these simple cooking techniques, I encourage you to waste no time in doing so. Getting more involved in the process of preparing food—and knowing what's in that food—is a key to long-term health.

The Technique . . . Steaming:

Chinese, Japanese, Singaporean, and Italian chefs all know how good—not to mention good for you—steamed foods can be. Steaming, which involves suspending the food in a closed pan above a hot liquid, preserves more nutrients than almost any other cooking method. I really encourage you to get into the swing of steaming. You won't regret it!

THE TOOLS

You might consider buying a steamer basket for about $10 at any house-wares store. This aluminum basket isn't just inexpensive; it takes up almost no room in the cabinet, and you can use it with just about any food. To use the basket, put a few inches of water in a pan, add the basket and then the veggies, and cover. In just a few minutes, you'll be able to enjoy perfectly cooked—and perfectly delicious—food.

You might also consider investing in an electric rice cooker if you want to steam your rice Japanese style. You can buy a basic model for about $30. Some of the more advanced models can be used not just for rice and veggies but also for fish, poultry, and other main course items.

The Technique . . . Stir-Frying:

Stir-frying involves cooking foods (usually small, cut-up pieces of meat and vegetables) over high heat with just a touch of added fat, usually in the form of olive or canola oil. Stir-frying is an excellent method for making tasty food fast.

THE TOOLS

Stir-frying is a cinch if you have the right wok. Pick up one of these large, round-bottomed pans—which Asian chefs rely on daily—to flash-fry foods without using a lot of oil. Woks are usually made of rolled steel, which makes it easy to control the cooking temperature. There are lots of great woks to choose from, but I recommend getting one with a nonstick surface to make cleanup easier.

If you don't feel like purchasing a wok just yet, you can shallow-fry foods in a large skillet. That's another great way to ease up on the oil without sacrificing any of the taste.

The Technique . . . Roasting:

Roasting is the French secret to meat and poultry perfection. A well-roasted dish is crisp on the outside and soft and chewy in the middle.

> ### And Don't Forget . . . Microwaving
>
> You heard me right—microwaving. Don't be afraid to take advantage of modern amenities like the microwave, which can steam all sorts of foods in a matter of minutes. But microwaves aren't just convenient tools for people with fast-paced lives. They can actually be good for your health, too. Because microwaves heat food so quickly and without any extra water, they often preserve more vitamins and minerals than other cooking methods. Microwaves also can expand your selection of healthy foods at the grocery store. There are a number of microwavable brown rices available that can be ready to eat in a minute. So don't feel as if you're "cheating" if you prepare your dinner in the microwave. Instead, focus on the more important thing—what's in that dinner. The microwave can be a great help on your journey to healthy living. If you know how to use it, you'll never have an excuse for not eating healthily!

Roasting is also a fast, delicious way to cook many different vegetables. To roast foods, you cook them uncovered in the oven on high heat. This is a very healthy way to prepare foods.

THE TOOLS

A roasting pan is a useful item to have on hand—and not just on Thanksgiving! I recommend a good-quality nonstick pan. And don't forget a roasting rack to place inside the pan. This allows the meat's fatty juices to drip down into the pan, which minimizes the amount of fat left in the meat you'll be serving. You can still use some of the drippings to make gravy, if you choose.

The Technique . . . Stewing:

The Spanish and Chinese love stewing, and so should you. It's the simple process of slow-cooking foods in a large, covered pot and is an efficient, straightforward technique for preparing meat and vegetables. Stewing is especially great for one-dish meals such as Spanish chickpea and spinach stew. The Japanese also make wonderful stews, including sukiyaki, one of my all-time favorite dishes.

Shortcuts

Don't be afraid of taking shortcuts in the kitchen. If you're in a hurry, pick up frozen or one-minute microwavable rice, or buy precooked or canned chicken to toss into salads and soups for added protein. Bags of frozen, precut, ready-to-stir-fry vegetables are also a great convenience. Canned beans and lentils can be an indispensable shortcut. There's no reason to soak legumes overnight unless you have the time and inclination. The end result is much more important than the process.

THE TOOLS

If you cook even occasionally, you probably have the only equipment you need to start stewing: a large ovenproof pot (with a lid) or Dutch oven.

SIXTEEN

The 5-Factor Lifestyle

Now that you understand all the new ingredients and cooking techniques we'll be working with, let's take a moment to consider one other factor that contributes to the health of my 5-Factor World Diet countries: lifestyle. Remember, my Top 10 countries share more than just a love of vegetables. They are also bound by culinary customs that help them put food in the proper perspective: as nourishment to be enjoyed and savored instead of just shoveled in. Let's take a look at the lessons we can learn from their traditions.

LESSON 1: TAKE YOUR TIME

I've said it before, and I'll probably say it again: Slowing down the pace of eating will not only make mealtimes more pleasant, it will also help with portion control and, over time, weight loss. From Spain to Israel, people linger over their meals for hours. And remarkably enough, even though the French and Italians are famous for their eight-course meals,

The Chopsticks Solution

Having trouble slowing down? Here's an idea: every once in a while, eat with chopsticks, as most Asians do. You don't have to be eating Asian food to use chopsticks. They're great for any food that doesn't require cutting.

Even if you're a high-speed eater, you might find that chopsticks, by their very design, will slow you down quite a bit. Rather than spearing a big piece of food with a fork or shoveling a massive amount into your mouth with a spoon, you can eat only what the chopsticks can hold. Check out EverythingChopsticks.com for all sorts of wonderful chopsticks for everyday use.

they often consume less food than we manage to cram onto a single plate! Longer, structured meals—the kind the French have made famous—are an excellent strategy both for adding variety to your meals and for controlling caloric intake. As a rule, a sense of satiety tends to lag behind your appetite: you can still be ravenous even when you've had more than enough to eat. If you can manage to stave off your appetite temporarily, a feeling of satisfaction will eventually follow. Pacing your meals is a good way to achieve this balance.

I'm the first to acknowledge that long sit-down dinners might not be possible in our hectic lives, but regardless of our commitments, we can all make an effort to slow down a little, to sit at a real table and eat off a real plate. Make a vow to stop eating on your feet or out of Styrofoam containers. And whenever possible, divide your meals into separate portions or courses so that you don't overstuff yourself. This is a great technique for both cutting back on the amount you eat and increasing your enjoyment of it.

Remember, eating is, or should be, an event. It should be more than mere "feeding."

LESSON 2: ENJOY YOURSELF

If you take more time with your meals, you might also find that you enjoy them more. In all my Top 10 countries, the food court is a recent—and unfortunate—innovation. For most people in the world, eating means gathering around a table with friends and loved ones, discussing what happened during the day. Eating is all about community and communal enjoyment.

Taking that extra bit of effort to "beautify" your meal is another way to increase the pleasure you take in it. Rather than scarf down fast food out of paper wrappers, the Japanese believe that the presentation is as important as the food itself. They go to great lengths to get every detail right, from the shape of the fish to the color of the pickled turnip. The Japanese also believe that food should stimulate all five senses, including sight, so try to make your meal colorful, with multiple ingredients from different food groups. This aesthetic consideration often results in boosting the nutritional profile of your meal at the same time.

The Japanese also serve meals on small side plates—the more decorative, the better. This trick not only makes the food more attractive, but it also serves the important dual purpose of cutting down on portion size and lengthening the duration of the meal.

LESSON 3: EVERYTHING IN MODERATION

Maintaining a healthy weight requires restricting portion size, and if there's one thread that links the World Diet countries, it's the belief in the fine art of moderation. From the Japanese discipline of *hara hachi bunme,* or eating until just 80 percent full, to the Swedish practice of *lagom,* or eating "just enough," people all over the planet know when to say when. The French, though famed for the richness of their food, make a point of not overeating. They would rather restrict their portion sizes than their selection of ingredients. The Spanish do the same, eating whatever they want—including heavy cheeses and cured pork—but always within limits.

LESSON 4: MIX IT UP

Striking the right balance of foods and flavors at every meal is a great way to keep your diet interesting, fun, and nutritious. Variety, as the type represented by the Swedish smorgasbord, really is the spice of life. The Japanese, Chinese, and Koreans have all adopted a version of the "five flavors" approach, meaning they try to incorporate all five flavors (bitter, sweet, spicy, salty, and sour) into every meal.

LESSON 5: GET CREATIVE

Having a good time, both when you're cooking and when you're eating, is essential to maintaining a healthy relationship with food—not to mention maintaining a healthy weight. Don't think of cooking as a chore, but as an exciting opportunity to exercise your creativity. When you're preparing food, don't let yourself be a slave to a recipe. As you get more confident in the kitchen, you'll be able to improvise more, like the Spanish do. Changing one or two ingredients in a dish might lead to unexpectedly delicious results.

Also as in other cultures, invite your kids into the kitchen and involve them in the process of preparing meals. Passing down recipes from one generation to the next is, or should be, an important part of every family's traditions, and it will also make your kitchen time livelier. You will impart valuable lessons to your kids and save yourself some work in the process!

LESSON 6: EXERCISE

Most cultures have a national sport. In my home country, Canada, it's hockey (and lacrosse). In the United States, it's baseball. In Italy, Spain, and many other European countries, it's football (soccer). The Japanese and Koreans practice martial arts such as karate and tae kwon do, and in China people of all ages gather in parks before dawn to perform tai chi. Swedes favor hiking through the forest and other hearty outdoor activities.

Although all of these pastimes are commendable (and often a lot of fun), they do not necessarily explain why people in some countries are so much fitter than those in others. When researching this book, I was struck time and again by the one thing that really seems to differentiate the healthy nations from the not-so-healthy ones: walking. People who walk more in their daily lives are in better shape, tend to weigh less, and live longer than people who are sedentary. On one level, it really is that simple. A recent Australian study found an inverse relationship between how much you weigh and how many steps you take each day, meaning that the more you walk, the less you weigh.

Our problem in the United States, and yet another big reason for our nationwide slide toward obesity, is that we just don't walk enough. Most of us take between 3,000 and 5,000 steps each day. But to be healthy, doctors recommend that we take twice that number, or roughly 10,000 steps, *every single day*. That's about five miles, which according to the U.S. surgeon general is the bare minimum to maintain cardiovascular health. Sometimes walking more is all that it takes to transform your life. You will sleep better, breathe better, and lose weight.

Easier said than done, right? Maybe not. The key thing to remember is that *every step counts*. You don't have to be sweating on a treadmill to be getting exercise. You can just be crossing the room to answer the phone or dashing outside to the mailbox.

There is an infinite number of ways to incorporate more walking into your day-to-day life. Try taking a pre- or post-dinner *passeggiata,* strolling around the neighborhood every evening before it gets dark. Or go on a Spanish-style paseo on Sunday to help digest your big meal of the week.

There are other ways you can increase the number of steps you walk every day, too. Leave your car at home every once in a while. Take public transportation instead—even if you have to walk fifteen minutes to the nearest station. In fact, the farther away from your house the station is, the more your body will thank you in the end. If you already take public transportation, leave for work a little early, get off at the station either before or after your destination, and walk the rest of the way. You might make some interesting discoveries about your city in the process.

If you don't live in an area with public transportation, carpool to work with a neighbor—and walk to your neighbor's to pick up your ride. (Then spend all that gas money you save on a new, smaller-size pair of jeans!) If you're a committed driver, choose the absolutely worst spot in the grocery store parking lot and walk the extra distance to and from your car. At the airport, skip the moving walkway and cover the distance between gates by walking. If you live or work in a building with an elevator, take the stairs instead—first just once a week, then maybe two or three times a week. (Many old buildings around the world aren't equipped with escalators and elevators, which forces people to take the

The Essential Advantages of "Active Transportation"

Walking for fitness is great, but walking for utility might have even bigger benefits. A recent study found that "active transportation"—or getting yourself where you need to go by walking or riding your bike—is a key factor in long-term health.[1] Americans, who have the lowest rate of active transportation among the countries in the study (only about 8 percent of us use active transportation to get to work), also have the highest obesity rate, while Europeans, who habitually walk or cycle to work, have the lowest obesity rate. Whereas Europeans do most of their daily errands on foot, we use cars for 55 percent of all trips that are half a kilometer in length and 85 percent of trips that are one kilometer.

I just can't overstate the importance of overcoming your dependence on a car (just a little) and fitting some low-impact, moderate-intensity exercise into your routine every day. To make my case, let me remind you of a remarkable statistic that I cited earlier in the book. The average European walks 237 miles every year and cycles 116 miles, while the average American walks 87 miles and cycles just 24 miles. The difference that makes in weight control is enormous, amounting to five to nine pounds of fat burned every year in Europe compared to just two pounds in the United States. Consider the impact of that difference over several years.

stairs—and tone their legs in the process.) If you work in an office setting, make the effort to walk across the room to communicate with your colleagues face-to-face. By making your lifestyle a little less efficient, you will make your body more efficient.

If you spend hours a day on the telephone at work or at home, invest in a headset and move around a little while you talk. You might even get some housework in! I promise that every single tiny bit of exercise you can sneak into your routine will have a big impact on your long-term health.

Even taken all together, these extra measures might not be enough for you to reach the 10,000-step goal. That's perfectly all right. First of all, you should try to improve your activity level gradually, over time. After a few weeks of increasing your daily steps, you could up the ante by taking a brisk walk around the neighborhood several mornings a

The Pedometer: A Step in the Right Direction

You might be shocked to learn how many steps you walk every day—and not in a good way. The best way to quantify exactly how much you walk is with a pedometer, a step-counting device that you can clip onto your belt or strap to your ankle. Studies have shown that wearing a pedometer can help increase people's awareness of their physical movements and then, with any luck, increase those movements. A Stanford University study found that people who wore pedometers increased their physical activity by 27 percent, or about 2,000 steps (one mile) every day.[2] They also lowered their body mass index (BMI).

Pedometers are inexpensive; a basic model can cost as little as $10. They're also lightweight and can fit in any purse or pocket. Wearing one can help you determine exactly how much you walk every day—and how much you *should* be walking. If you wear a pedometer, try to keep a daily log of your mileage and track your improvement over time. Your progress will inspire you to keep moving.

week. Find a walking buddy (or a loaded iPod) to make these journeys more fun. Or bring a comfortable pair of shoes to work and spend part of every lunch hour strolling around. If you want to step it up a notch and really start shedding the pounds, try to go beyond the 10,000-step baseline goal and walk up to 15,000 steps a day.

There are so many simple activities you can do to make your lifestyle a little healthier. One study found that women who walked at a moderate pace for as little as one hour a week significantly cut their risk of heart disease.[3] Regular walking also has been shown to reduce blood pressure, lower the risk of diabetes and stroke, and increase lung capacity. Inactivity is a leading contributor to chronic health problems, so the more you move, the healthier you'll be.

———

Has all this talk of exercise got your appetite up? If so, that's excellent. Because at long last, it's time for you to dig into some of the healthiest—and most delicious—recipes on the planet.

PART 4

THE 5-FACTOR
WORLD DIET RECIPES

Miso Soup with Tofu

SERVES 2

PREP TIME: 5 MINUTES • COOK TIME: 15 MINUTES

Miso can be found in Japanese markets and the refrigerated section of many supermarkets. It comes in different varieties. Here the milder, lighter-colored variety is used. If you can find it, use low-fat tofu.

TIP: Check out instant miso soup mixes, now available in some markets. Just add water for the quickest Asian-style breakfast ever.

1 can (14½ ounces) reduced-sodium chicken broth

2 tablespoons light-colored miso paste

1 tablespoon mirin or rice vinegar

½ cup frozen green peas, thawed

¾ cup diced firm silken tofu

1 scallion, thinly sliced

1–1½ cups cooked brown rice, warmed

Warm 1 cup of the broth in a small saucepan over medium heat. Stir in the miso paste. Cook for 3 minutes, mashing the paste against the side of the pot to help dissolve it. Add the remaining broth, 1 cup water, and the mirin; bring to a boil. Reduce the heat and simmer for 6 minutes. Add the peas and cook for 2 minutes more.

Add the tofu. Remove the pot from the heat and let sit for 3 minutes. Ladle the soup into 2 bowls and garnish with the scallion. Serve with the rice on the side, adding it to the bowl, if desired.

Soba Noodle Bowl
with Cucumber and Cabbage

SERVES 2

PREP TIME: 5 MINUTES • COOK TIME: 5 MINUTES

In Japan, soba noodles are served hot and cold, for breakfast, lunch, and dinner. If you can't find them, substitute whole wheat spaghetti.

> 1 tablespoon reduced-sodium soy sauce
>
> 1 tablespoon rice vinegar
>
> 1 tablespoon fresh lemon juice
>
> 1 teaspoon sesame or vegetable oil
>
> 4 ounces soba or udon noodles
>
> 1 cooked boneless, skinless chicken breast half (about 4 ounces), diced or
>   shredded
>
> 2 scallions, thinly sliced
>
> 1 cucumber or ½ English cucumber, peeled, seeded, and thinly sliced
>
> 1 cup coleslaw mix

In a small bowl, whisk the soy sauce, vinegar, lemon juice, and oil until well blended.

Cook the noodles according to the package directions. Drain and rinse under cold water until cool.

In a large bowl, combine the noodles, chicken, scallions, cucumber, and coleslaw mix. Toss with the soy dressing and serve.

LUNCH

Soba Noodle Stir-Fry

SERVES 2

PREP TIME: 10 MINUTES • COOK TIME: 20 MINUTES

Quick-cooking soba noodles are made from buckwheat, which means they provide more fiber than wheat or rice noodles.

3 ounces soba noodles

4 ounces extra-firm tofu, drained, patted dry, and cut into small cubes

Salt

1 stalk broccoli, cut into small florets, stems thinly sliced

2 ounces sugar snap peas

1 tablespoon reduced-fat smooth peanut butter

1 tablespoon rice vinegar

1 tablespoon reduced-sodium soy sauce

Pinch of red pepper flakes, if desired

2 cloves garlic, minced

Cook the noodles according to the package directions. Drain and rinse well under cold water to prevent sticking.

Lightly coat a large nonstick skillet with cooking spray; place over medium-high heat. Add the tofu and season with salt. Cook for 8 minutes, until golden, stirring occasionally. Transfer to a platter.

Coat the skillet again with cooking spray; place over medium-high heat. Add the broccoli, peas, and a splash of water. Cover and cook for 5 minutes, until the vegetables are crisp-tender.

Meanwhile, make the sauce. In a small bowl, whisk together the peanut butter and 2 tablespoons water. Whisk in the vinegar, soy sauce, and pepper flakes, if desired.

Add the reserved noodles, the tofu, garlic, and sauce to the vegetables. Cook for 2 minutes, tossing, until the noodles are warmed through. Serve.

Fried Rice with Mushrooms and Edamame

SERVES 2

PREP TIME: 10 MINUTES • COOK TIME: 7 MINUTES

You'll find cooked brown rice and shelled edamame beans in the frozen food section of health food stores and supermarkets. Instant brown rice is another quick option.

Salt and black pepper

1 egg white, lightly beaten

$\frac{1}{3}$ pound shiitake mushrooms, stemmed, wiped clean, and thinly sliced

$\frac{3}{4}$ cup frozen shelled edamame, thawed

2 cloves garlic, minced

1 cup cooked brown rice

4 scallions, thinly sliced on the diagonal

3 tablespoons fresh lime juice

1 tablespoon reduced-sodium soy sauce

Coat a large nonstick skillet with cooking spray; place over medium heat. Whisk salt and pepper to taste into the egg white. Add to the skillet; cook without stirring for 1 minute, until set. Run a rubber spatula around the pan to release the cooked egg and slide it onto a cutting board. Roll up and thinly slice crosswise.

Coat the skillet again with cooking spray; place over medium heat. Add the mushrooms, edamame, and garlic; cook for 4 minutes, until the mushrooms are tender, stirring often. Stir in the rice, egg slices, scallions, lime juice, and soy sauce. Cook for 2 minutes, tossing, until the rice is warmed through. Serve.

SNACKS

Smoked Salmon Nori Roll

SERVES 2

PREP TIME: 10 MINUTES

To stick with the 5-Factor program, I use brown rice for this sushi. Brown rice doesn't stick together in the same way sushi rice does, so the roll may be harder to work with.

1½ cups cooked brown rice

1 tablespoon rice vinegar

2 teaspoons reduced-sodium soy sauce, plus more for serving

2 sheets nori (dried seaweed)

4 ounces sliced smoked salmon, cut into strips

½ cup snow peas, trimmed and very thinly sliced lengthwise

2 tablespoons fresh lemon juice, divided

In a medium bowl, combine the rice, vinegar, and soy sauce.

To make the rolls, place a bamboo sushi mat on the countertop with the slats running crosswise. Lay a sheet of nori on the mat, shiny side down. Lightly moisten your hands; spread half of the rice on the nori, leaving a 1½-inch border on each long side. Place half of the salmon strips in a horizontal line across the middle of the rice. Place half of the snow pea strips in a horizontal line above the salmon. Drizzle 1 tablespoon lemon juice over the rice.

Beginning with the edge nearest to you, lift the mat up with your thumbs, holding the filling in place with your fingers, and fold the mat over the filling so that the upper and lower edges of the rice meet. Squeeze gently but firmly along the length of the roll and tug the top edge of the mat away from you to tighten. Using both hands, press the roll firmly inside the bamboo roller. Transfer the roll to a plate, cover with a damp, clean kitchen towel, and place in the refrigerator. Repeat with the remaining sheet of nori and ingredients.

Remove the rolls from the refrigerator. Dip a sharp knife in water; cut each roll into 8 equal pieces. Serve with soy sauce.

Spicy Tuna Sushi Roll

SERVES 2

PREP TIME: 10 MINUTES

When making tuna sushi, it's vital that the fish be as fresh as possible, since it is not cooked.

TIP: Sushi rice is traditionally used when making sushi. Unfortunately, it is very low in fiber, so I suggest switching to brown rice.

1½ cups cooked brown rice

1 tablespoon rice vinegar

2 teaspoons reduced-sodium soy sauce, plus more for serving

2 sheets nori (dried seaweed)

4 ounces sushi-grade yellowfin tuna, cut into ¾-inch-wide strips

2 teaspoons wasabi paste

Cook the rice according to the package directions.

In a medium bowl, combine the rice, vinegar, and soy sauce.

To make the rolls, place a bamboo sushi mat on the countertop with the slats running crosswise. Lay a sheet of nori on the mat, shiny side down. Lightly moisten your hands; spread half of the rice on the nori, leaving a 1½-inch border on each long side. Place half of the tuna strips in a horizontal line across the middle of the rice. Place half of the wasabi paste in a horizontal line above the tuna.

Beginning with the edge nearest to you, lift the mat up with your thumbs, holding the filling in place with your fingers, and fold the mat over the filling so that the upper and lower edges of the rice meet. Squeeze gently but firmly along the length of the roll and tug the top edge of the mat away from you to tighten. Using both hands, press the roll firmly inside the bamboo roller. Transfer the roll to a plate, cover with a damp towel, and place in the refrigerator. Repeat with the remaining sheet of nori and ingredients.

Remove the rolls from the refrigerator. Dip a sharp knife in water; cut each roll into 8 equal pieces. Serve with soy sauce.

Fresh Vegetable Hand Roll

SERVES 2

PREP TIME: 10 MINUTES

Mirin is a widely used sauce in Japanese cooking. It is a type of sweet-ened rice wine similar to sake but without the high alcohol content.

1½ cups cooked brown rice

1 tablespoon mirin or rice vinegar

2 sheets nori (dried seaweed)

3 ounces frozen cooked (peeled and deveined) shrimp, chopped

½ carrot, peeled and cut into ¼-by-3-inch matchsticks

½ red bell pepper, cut into ¼-by-3-inch matchsticks

1 scallion, cut into ¼-by-3-inch matchsticks

Wasabi paste

Reduced-sodium soy sauce

In a medium bowl, combine the rice and mirin.

To make the rolls, place a bamboo sushi mat on the countertop with the slats running crosswise. Lay a sheet of nori on the mat, shiny side down. Lightly moisten your hands; spread half of the rice on the nori, leaving a 1½-inch border on each long side. Place half of the shrimp and carrot sticks in 2 horizontal lines across the middle of the rice. Make similar horizontal lines of pepper and scallion sticks.

Beginning with the edge nearest to you, lift the mat up with your thumbs, holding the filling in place with your fingers, and fold the mat over the filling so that the upper and lower edges of the rice meet. Squeeze gently but firmly along the length of the roll and tug the top edge of the mat away from you to tighten. Using both hands, press the roll firmly inside the bamboo roller. Transfer the roll to a plate, cover with a damp towel, and place in the refrigerator. Repeat with the remaining sheet of nori and ingredients. Remove rolls from refrigerator. Dip a sharp knife in water; cut each roll into 8 equal pieces. Serve with soy sauce.

Chicken Yakatori

SERVES 2

PREP TIME: 5 MINUTES (PLUS MARINATING) • COOK TIME: 6 MINUTES

TIP: If you are using wooden skewers, soak them in water for at least 10 minutes before assembling the kebabs to prevents scorching. For ease of cooking, thread the chicken strips on the skewers so that they lay as flat as possible.

¼ cup mirin

¼ cup reduced-sodium soy sauce

1 tablespoon agave nectar

2 tablespoons rice vinegar

1 teaspoon peeled and minced fresh ginger

2 boneless, skinless chicken breast halves (about 4 ounces each), cut into thick strips

1 red bell pepper, thickly sliced

2 scallions, each cut into 8 pieces

1½ cups cooked brown rice, warmed

In a small saucepan, warm the mirin, soy sauce, agave nectar, vinegar, and ginger until the agave is dissolved.

Thread the chicken, pepper, and scallions on 8 wooden or metal skewers. Place the 8- to 10-inch skewers in a 9-by-13-inch glass baking dish and drench with the sauce. Let marinate for 30 minutes.

Preheat the grill or a nonstick grill pan over heat. Add the skewers; grill for 3 minutes per side, until the chicken is cooked through, turning occasionally and brushing with marinade during the first 3 minutes of cooking. Serve the skewers atop the warm rice.

Iced Raspberry Green Tea

SERVES 2

PREP TIME: 5 MINUTES

We've taken the traditional green tea of Japan and turned it into a super-cooling iced drink—a fantastically refreshing snack on a hot day. A bonus: each serving contains more than half your daily dose of vitamin C.

TIP: Whey protein powder is preferred, but soy protein powder is another option.

1½ cups frozen raspberries

¾ cup brewed green tea, at room temperature or cold

1½ scoops whey protein powder

1 tablespoon agave nectar

1 tablespoon fresh lime juice

Seltzer water

Lime wedges

In a blender or food processor, combine the berries and tea; purée until blended. Add the protein powder, agave nectar, and lime juice; process until smooth and frothy. Pour over ice in two tall glasses. Top off with a splash of seltzer and garnish with lime wedges.

DINNER

Grilled Sesame-Orange Tuna

SERVES 2

PREP TIME: 10 MINUTES • COOK TIME: 5 MINUTES

No time at all? Substitute ¼ cup prepared sesame-ginger vinaigrette for the homemade marinade.

Marinade

2 tablespoons orange juice

½ teaspoon canola or vegetable oil

1 tablespoon rice vinegar

1 small clove garlic, minced

1 teaspoon grated orange zest

½ teaspoon Asian sesame oil

Salt and black pepper

2 tuna fillets (about 5 ounces each)

4 ounces green beans, trimmed

4 cups mizuna or other small green lettuce leaves

1½ cups cooked brown rice, warmed

To make the marinade, in a glass or plastic measuring cup, whisk all the ingredients.

Place the tuna in a nonreactive baking dish, pour the marinade over the fish, and turn to coat. Marinate, refrigerated, for 30 minutes.

Preheat the grill or a grill pan over medium-high heat; lightly coat with cooking spray. Remove the fish from the marinade (discard the marinade); grill for 3 minutes. Carefully turn the fish; grill for 2 minutes, until browned yet still translucent on the inside.

Meanwhile, steam the green beans until just crisp-tender.

Arrange the mizuna on a serving platter; top with the beans and fish. Serve with the rice.

Salmon Teriyaki with Asian Coleslaw

SERVES 2

PREP TIME: 5 MINUTES • COOK TIME: 15 MINUTES

Deep-sea fish such as salmon tend to be a great source of omega-3 fatty acids and thus carry more fat than freshwater fish. Remember, these are heart-healthy fats—good fats to include in your diet.

TIP: You can make the super-quick coleslaw up to 4 hours in advance.

¼ cup reduced-sodium soy sauce

2 tablespoons mirin

2 tablespoons agave nectar

1 tablespoon peeled and minced fresh ginger

1 tablespoon minced garlic

2 salmon fillets (about 4 ounces each)

4 ounces soba noodles, cooked (warm or cold)

Asian Coleslaw (see below)

In a small saucepan over medium-low heat, bring the soy sauce, mirin, agave nectar, ginger, and garlic to a simmer. Reduce the heat and simmer for 5 to 7 minutes, until the mixture thickens, stirring often.

Place the salmon in a resealable plastic bag, add the marinade, and turn to coat. Refrigerate for at least 30 minutes or up to 3 hours.

Preheat the oven to 400°F. Lightly coat a medium ovenproof skillet with cooking spray; set over medium-high heat. Cook the salmon for 4 minutes. Turn the fish, transfer the skillet to the oven, and cook for 4 minutes, until cooked through.

Serve the salmon atop the noodles, with the coleslaw on the side.

Asian Coleslaw: In a medium bowl, whisk 2 tablespoons light mayonnaise, 2 tablespoons fresh lemon juice, and ½ teaspoon Asian sesame oil. Fold in 1½ cups coleslaw mix until coated. Garnish with 2 tablespoons sliced scallions and season with salt and pepper. Refrigerate for at least 30 minutes. Serve chilled.

Shabu-Shabu

SERVES 2

PREP TIME: 10 MINUTES • COOK TIME: VARIES

Shabu-shabu means swishing your dinner ingredients back and forth in boiling broth to cook them. The broth can be eaten as a soup after the meat is eaten.

> 8 ounces flank steak or sirloin, very thinly sliced
>
> 4 shiitake mushrooms, stemmed, wiped clean, and cut in half if large
>
> 1 cup shredded Chinese (napa) cabbage
>
> ½ cup grated daikon
>
> 6 cups chicken broth
>
> 1–1½ cups cooked brown rice, warmed
>
> Soy-Ginger Dipping Sauce (see below)

Arrange the meat slices and vegetables separately on 2 platters.

Pour the broth into a medium saucepan; bring to a boil over medium-high heat. Using chopsticks, pick up the meat and vegetables and swish back and forth in the boiling broth until cooked to the desired doneness. Serve with the rice and dipping sauce.

Soy-Ginger Dipping Sauce: In a small bowl, whisk ¼ cup reduced-sodium soy sauce, 2 tablespoons mirin, 2 tablespoons rice vinegar, 1 teaspoon peeled and minced fresh ginger, and a pinch of red pepper flakes.

Smooth Peach-Raspberry Lassi

SERVES 2

PREP TIME: 3 MINUTES

Lassi is a cool South Asian drink traditionally made with yogurt, honey, and mangoes. We've substituted orange juice and always-available frozen peaches and raspberries here.

1 cup frozen peaches

½ cup frozen raspberries

¼ cup nonfat plain yogurt

2 tablespoons orange juice

4-6 ice cubes

In a blender or food processor, purée the peaches, raspberries, yogurt, and orange juice until smooth. Add the ice; process until the ice is crushed and the drink is frothy. Pour into glasses and serve.

Coconut Spinach Cup

SERVES 2

PREP TIME: 5 MINUTES • COOK TIME: 20 MINUTES

Most South Asians eat savory dishes for breakfast, like this richly satisfying and super-nutritious rice dish. We've added spinach for color and a blast of vitamin A.

½ cup instant brown rice

Unsweetened light coconut milk (check rice package directions for amount)

Salt to taste

5 ounces baby spinach

2 cloves garlic, minced

½ cup frozen shelled edamame, thawed

In a small saucepan, combine the rice and coconut milk, substituting the coconut milk for the water called for on the package. Cook approximately 20 minutes according to the package directions, uncovering the pot to check on the rice a few times while cooking. Add more coconut milk if the rice dries out.

Lightly coat a medium saucepan with cooking spray; place over medium-low heat. Gradually add the spinach to the pot, stirring often. Add the garlic and edamame. Continue to cook, stirring, until the spinach is wilted, about 5 minutes. Serve the spinach atop the warm rice, adding salt to taste.

Curried Sweet Potato with Warm Paratha Bread

SERVES 2

PREP TIME: 5 MINUTES • COOK TIME: 17 MINUTES

Sweet potato curry puffs are a popular Singaporean street food. Slather this luscious curry-spiked sweet potato purée on warm whole-grain paratha bread if you can find it. If not, use whole-grain pita bread instead.

½ small onion, diced

½–1 teaspoon red curry paste, to taste

½ teaspoon ground cumin

¼ teaspoon ground cinnamon

1 large sweet potato (about 10 ounces), unpeeled, cut into small dice

¾ cup nonfat milk, or more as needed

½ cup nonfat plain yogurt

2 teaspoons fresh lime juice

Salt and black pepper

2 whole-grain paratha breads, warmed

Coat a medium nonstick skillet with cooking spray; place over medium-low heat. Add the onion; cook for 2 minutes, until softened, stirring. Add the curry paste, cumin, and cinnamon; cook for 30 seconds, stirring to dissolve the paste. Add the sweet potato; cook for 2 minutes, stirring to coat.

Pour in the milk. Simmer for 12 minutes, until the sweet potato is tender, stirring often and adding more milk if the mixture dries out.

Transfer to a food processor or blender. Add the yogurt and lime juice; process until smooth. Season with salt and pepper. Serve with the warm bread.

Cool Lemongrass Chicken and Rice Salad

SERVES 2

PREP TIME: 10 MINUTES • COOK TIME: 3 MINUTES

Lemongrass is a lemon-scented plant widely used in Southeast Asian cooking. To add it to dishes, use a very sharp knife to slice through the yellow section of the stalk, then pound the slices to release the flavor. Since lemongrass can be stringy, it needs to be puréed in a food processor or cooked until softened.

TIP: If lemongrass is unavailable, substitute grated lemon zest.

1 teaspoon canola oil

1 stalk lemongrass, chopped, or 1 teaspoon grated lemon zest

1 small red chile, seeded and chopped

2 scallions, sliced

1 cup cooked brown rice

1 tablespoon fresh lime juice

1 teaspoon fish sauce

1 cup shredded cooked chicken breast

½ cup finely chopped fresh mint

Warm the oil in a medium nonstick skillet over medium heat. Add the lemongrass, chile, and scallions; cook for 3 minutes, until softened, stirring. Fold in the cooked rice until coated.

In a medium serving bowl, whisk the lime juice and fish sauce. Fold in the rice mixture, then the chicken and mint. Refrigerate until ready to serve.

Mee Goreng (Singapore Noodles)

SERVES 2

PREP TIME: 10 MINUTES • COOK TIME: 10 MINUTES

If you can't find mustard greens, use spinach in this traditional Singaporean stir-fry.

4 ounces mustard greens, washed, thick stems discarded

4 ounces soba or wide rice noodles

2 tablespoons reduced-sodium soy sauce

1 teaspoon Asian hot chili paste or sauce, such as sambal oelek

1 teaspoon canola oil

2 tablespoons peeled and minced fresh ginger

1 cup canned diced tomatoes, drained

8 ounces precooked (peeled and deveined) medium shrimp, fresh or frozen

4 ounces bean sprouts

¼ cup chopped fresh cilantro

Lime wedges

Bring a large pot of salted water to a boil. Add the mustard greens; cook for 30 seconds. Lift the greens out of the pot with tongs and set in a strainer to drain.

Add the noodles to the boiling water in the pot; cook according to the package directions. Drain and rinse with cold water.

In a small bowl, combine the soy sauce and chili paste; set aside.

Warm the oil in a large nonstick skillet over medium heat. Add the ginger; cook for 30 seconds, stirring. Add the tomatoes; cook for 2 minutes, stirring. Add the shrimp and blanched greens; cook for 3 minutes, stirring. Add the noodles and soy sauce mixture; cook until warmed through. Add the bean sprouts and cilantro. Serve with lime wedges.

SNACK

Indian-Spiced Chickpea and Chicken Bowl

SERVES 2

PREP TIME: 10 MINUTES • COOK TIME: 3 MINUTES

In spite of the number of ingredients, this meal can be ready in less than 15 minutes. Save time by using precooked chicken breast, perhaps from a rotisserie chicken.

1 stalk lemongrass, chopped, or 1 teaspoon grated lemon zest (see page 144).

1 clove garlic, minced

½ teaspoon Asian sesame oil

½ teaspoon curry powder

1 teaspoon peeled and minced fresh ginger

2 tablespoons chopped shallot

Salt and black pepper

⅔ cup canned chickpeas, drained and rinsed

½ cup shredded cooked chicken breast

2 tablespoons chopped fresh cilantro

Lemon wedges

Lightly coat a medium nonstick skillet with cooking spray; set over medium heat. Add the lemongrass, garlic, sesame oil, curry powder, ginger, shallot, and salt and pepper to taste. Cook for 1 minute to combine the flavors and toast the spices. Add the chickpeas and chicken; cook for 2 minutes to warm through, stirring often.

Spoon the mixture into 2 small bowls. Garnish each with 1 tablespoon cilantro. Serve with lemon wedges.

Shrimp and Noodle Stir-Fry

SERVES 2

PREP TIME: 5 MINUTES • COOK TIME: 10 MINUTES

Frozen shrimp are a must-have for quick meals. Not only are the shrimp already peeled and deveined, but they are usually precooked as well. We use high-fiber soba noodles to increase the fiber.

2 ounces soba or udon noodles

½ red chile, seeded and chopped

2 large cloves garlic, minced

3 ounces frozen precooked (peeled and deveined) medium-size shrimp, thawed

1 head baby bok choy, cored and thinly shredded, or 4 ounces spinach, shredded

2 tablespoons frozen green peas, thawed

1 tablespoon reduced-sodium soy sauce

1 tablespoon sweet chili sauce

Cook the noodles according to the package directions; drain.

Coat a large nonstick skillet with cooking spray; place over medium-high heat. Add the chile and garlic; cook for 1 minute, stirring. Add the shrimp, bok choy, and peas; cook for 3 minutes, stirring. Add the noodles, soy sauce, and chili sauce; cook to warm through. Serve.

Curried Chicken Wontons

MAKES 18 WONTONS

PREP TIME: 15 MINUTES • COOK TIME: 20 MINUTES

Curry is one of the most common flavors found in Singaporean food. Adjust the amount of curry paste used here according to your taste.

½ cup shredded carrots

1 cup shredded mustard greens or spinach

¼–½ teaspoon red curry paste, to taste

2 ounces ground chicken breast

¼ teaspoon curry powder

2 scallions, thinly sliced

Salt

1 egg white, lightly beaten

18 wonton wrappers

Coat a medium nonstick skillet with cooking spray; place over medium heat. Add the carrots and greens; cook for 4 minutes, until softened and wilted. Stir in the curry paste and 2 tablespoons water; cook for 30 seconds, until all the curry paste is absorbed. Stir in the chicken, curry powder, scallions, and salt to taste. Remove from the heat; stir in the egg white.

Hold a wonton wrapper in your palm. Place 1 rounded teaspoon of filling slightly off-center in the wrapper. Fold one side of the wrapper over the filling. Using your thumb and index finger, seal the wonton by pinching the wrapper together.

Coat a large nonstick skillet with cooking spray and set over medium-high heat. Add the wontons; cook for 4 minutes, until golden on the bottom. Turn and cook for 2 minutes. Reduce the heat to low, add ½ cup water to the skillet, and cover immediately. Cook for 4 minutes, covered, until most of the water is absorbed and the wontons are slightly translucent. Uncover, increase the heat to medium-high, and cook for 4 minutes, without stirring, until the bottoms are browned and crisp. Transfer to a paper-towel-lined plate to drain. Serve.

Spicy Dahl

SERVES 4

PREP TIME: 10 MINUTES • COOK TIME: 37 MINUTES

Dahl is a lentil-based dip or side dish. Save this snack for multiple meals:
It will keep for a week in your refrigerator, tightly sealed.

1 small onion, minced

4 cloves garlic, minced

1 tablespoon peeled and grated fresh ginger

½ teaspoon chili powder

½ teaspoon ground cumin

¼ teaspoon ground cinnamon

1 teaspoon salt

1 cup dried green or red lentils, washed and picked over

2 tablespoons tomato paste

4 cups vegetable broth or water

1 tablespoon fresh lime juice

¼ cup chopped fresh cilantro

Coat a medium saucepan with cooking spray; place over medium-high
heat. Add the onion; cook for 5 minutes, stirring. Add the garlic and
ginger; cook for 2 minutes, stirring. Add the chili powder, cumin, cinnamon, and salt; cook for 2 minutes, stirring.

Add the lentils, tomato paste, and broth. Bring to a boil; reduce the
heat and simmer for 20 minutes. Add water if the mixture dries out too
much.

Add the lime juice and cilantro; simmer for 8 minutes, until the
lentils are tender. Serve warm or at room temperature.

DINNER

Ginger Beef and Noodles

SERVES 2

PREP TIME: 5 MINUTES • COOK TIME: 10 MINUTES

Hoisin sauce, a prepared mixture of fermented soybeans, red rice, and spices, is a versatile condiment that offers sweetness with a slight kick to stir-fries.

4 ounces udon or thick rice noodles

2 tablespoons hoisin sauce

2 tablespoons reduced-sodium chicken broth

½ teaspoon canola or sesame oil

8 ounces flank steak, very thinly sliced

1 stalk broccoli, cut into small florets, stems thinly sliced

1 tablespoon peeled and minced fresh ginger

¼ cup thinly sliced scallions

Cook the noodles according to the package directions; drain.

In a small bowl, combine the hoisin sauce and broth.

Warm the oil in a large nonstick skillet over medium-high heat. Add the steak; cook for 4 minutes, stirring to brown both sides. Remove the meat to a platter. Add the broccoli and ¼ cup water to the pan; cover and cook for 3 minutes. Add the ginger; cook for 1 minute, stirring constantly. Stir in the meat, noodles, and hoisin mixture; cook to warm through and coat the noodles. Garnish with the scallions and serve.

Seared Sesame Scallops in Noodle Broth

SERVES 2

PREP TIME: 2 MINUTES (PLUS MARINATING) • COOK TIME: 10 MIN-
UTES

Asian, or toasted, sesame oil is a rich, strongly flavored oil that is used as
a seasoning only, not in cooking. You don't need much to impart a nutty
taste to any dish.

1 teaspoon Asian sesame oil

1 tablespoon reduced-sodium soy sauce

6 ounces sea scallops (about 6)

4 ounces somen or udon noodles

4 ounces snow peas, trimmed

1 cup vegetable or reduced-sodium chicken broth, warmed

2 scallions, thinly sliced

In a medium bowl, combine the sesame oil and soy sauce. Add the scallops; turn to coat. Marinate for 10 minutes.

Cook the noodles according to the package directions. Add the snow
peas in the last 2 minutes of the cooking time. Drain.

Coat a medium nonstick skillet with cooking spray; set over
medium-high heat. Add the scallops; cook for 2 to 3 minutes per side.

Arrange the noodles and peas in 2 deep serving bowls. Divide the
broth between the bowls. Top with the scallops, garnish with the scallions, and serve.

Tandoori Chicken with Cool Raita

SERVES 2

PREP TIME: 10 MINUTES • COOK TIME: 12 MINUTES

Although tandoori chicken is usually cooked in a superhot oven, home cooks should cook over a lower flame, or the creamy yogurt sauce will burn. Serve with hearty lentils and raita, a refreshing cucumber and yogurt condiment.

TIP: Garam masala is a blend of ground spices commonly used in Indian cooking.

2 boneless, skinless chicken breast halves (about 4 ounces each)

$^3/_4$ cup nonfat plain Greek yogurt

3 teaspoons fresh lemon juice, divided

1 teaspoon ground cumin

$^1/_2$ teaspoon paprika

$^1/_2$ teaspoon ground turmeric

$^1/_2$ teaspoon garam masala

Salt and black pepper

1 cup canned lentils, drained and rinsed

Cool Raita (see page 153)

With a sharp knife, make three slashes crosswise on the top of each chicken breast half.

In a medium nonreactive bowl, combine the yogurt, 1 teaspoon of the lemon juice, the cumin, paprika, turmeric, garam masala, and salt and pepper to taste. Add the chicken and turn to coat. Cover and refrigerate for at least 1 hour or overnight.

Preheat the grill or a grill pan over medium-high heat. Remove the chicken from the bowl; discard the marinade. Grill the chicken for 6 minutes per side, until cooked through.

In a small bowl, toss the lentils with the remaining 2 teaspoons lemon juice and salt and pepper to taste. Divide the lentils between 2 serving plates and top with the chicken. Serve with the raita.

Spiced Chai Tea Smoothie

SERVES 1

PREP TIME: 5 MINUTES

This is our cool version of the spiced milky tea served throughout South Asia. If you use vanilla yogurt, you can omit the agave nectar. Serve with whole wheat toast to add fiber to the meal.

¼ cup nonfat milk

2 chai tea bags

1 tablespoon agave nectar

¼ cup nonfat plain or vanilla yogurt

1 scoop whey protein powder

6–8 ice cubes

Ground cinnamon

Pour the milk into a mug; warm in the microwave until hot. Add the tea bags; steep for 10 minutes. Discard the tea bags, stir in the agave nectar, and place the mug in the freezer for 5 minutes.

In a blender or food processor, purée the chai milk mixture and yogurt. Add the protein powder and ice; process until the ice is crushed and the drink is frothy. Pour into a glass, sprinkle with cinnamon, and serve.

Cool Raita: Grate ½ peeled English cucumber into a medium colander set in the sink. Using a clean kitchen towel, squeeze the cucumber to release any excess moisture. In a small bowl, combine the cucumber, 1 cup nonfat plain Greek yogurt, 2 tablespoons chopped fresh mint, 1 teaspoon fresh lemon juice, and salt to taste. Refrigerate until serving.

BREAKFAST

Spiced Rice Congee with Pear

SERVES 1

PREP TIME: 2 MINUTES • COOK TIME: 18 MINUTES

Congee, or rice porridge, is a typical breakfast throughout China. If available, try topping it with Asian pear slices.

⅓ cup short-grain rice

2 cups nonfat milk

½ teaspoon ground cinnamon

½ teaspoon vanilla extract

Pinch of salt

1 medium pear, cored and sliced

In a small saucepan over medium heat, combine the rice and milk. Add the cinnamon, vanilla, and salt; bring to a low simmer. Cook for 18 minutes, stirring often, until the rice is very soft. Transfer to a serving bowl, top with the pear slices, and serve.

Crisp Scallion and Rice Omelet

SERVES 2

PREP TIME: 5 MINUTES   •   COOK TIME: 11 MINUTES

Increase the spiciness of this savory rice omelet by adding more fresh chiles or a dash of hot sauce.

TIP: Use frozen or microwavable brown rice to save time.

1 cup cooked brown rice

2 scallions, thinly sliced

1 small red chile, seeded and minced

½ cup frozen shelled edamame, thawed

3 egg whites

1 whole egg

Salt to taste

Reduced-sodium soy sauce

Preheat the oven to 350°F. Lightly coat a medium ovenproof nonstick skillet with cooking spray; place over medium-high heat. Add the rice; cook for 3 minutes, until toasted, stirring. Add the scallions, chile, and edamame; cook for 2 minutes, stirring.

In a medium bowl, lightly whisk the egg whites, whole egg, and salt. Transfer to the hot pan, spreading evenly. Cook, without stirring, for 3 minutes. Place the skillet in the oven for 3 minutes, until the eggs have set.

Run a spatula around the edge of the pan and slide the omelet onto a plate. Serve with soy sauce.

LUNCH

Chow Mein for Two

SERVES 2

PREP TIME: 5 MINUTES • COOK TIME: 7 MINUTES

The Chinese strive for the harmony of five flavors—salty, sweet, sour, spicy, and bitter—in their food. This colorful stir-fry achieves this goal.

TIP: If you can find low-fat tofu (less than one-third of its calories from fat), use it.

3 ounces thin rice noodles (vermicelli)

2 tablespoons reduced-sodium soy sauce

1 tablespoon oyster sauce

1 teaspoon Asian sesame oil

1 small red bell pepper, thinly sliced

2 ounces green beans, trimmed and cut in half lengthwise

4 ounces extra-firm tofu, drained, patted dry, and diced

2 teaspoons peeled and minced fresh ginger

Cook the noodles according to the package directions. Drain and rinse under cold water to prevent sticking.

In a small bowl, combine the soy sauce, oyster sauce, sesame oil, and 2 tablespoons water.

Lightly coat a large nonstick skillet with cooking spray; place over medium-high heat.

Add the pepper and beans; stir-fry for 2 minutes. Add the tofu; cook for 4 minutes, stirring. Add the ginger; stir-fry for 1 minute. Add the noodles and sauce mixture; cook, stirring, until combined and warmed through. Serve.

Egg Drop Soup with Fresh Spinach

SERVES 2

PREP TIME: 5 MINUTES • COOK TIME: 5 MINUTES

Serve this classic quick soup with brown rice crackers to increase the fiber and for dipping.

2 cups reduced-sodium chicken broth

3 ounces baby spinach, thinly sliced

3 scallions, thinly sliced on the diagonal

4 ounces shiitake mushrooms, stemmed, wiped clean, and thinly sliced

1 teaspoon reduced-sodium soy sauce

2 egg whites, lightly beaten

Asian sesame oil

8 brown rice crackers

In a medium saucepan over high heat, bring the chicken broth and 2 cups water to a simmer. Add the spinach, scallions, mushrooms, and soy sauce; cook for 1 minute, stirring.

Very slowly pour the egg whites into the pot; immediately turn off the heat. Use a fork to stir the egg whites in a clockwise direction to make thin ribbons in the broth. Ladle into 2 bowls and garnish each with a drop of sesame oil. Serve with the crackers.

Crispy Spiced Chicken

SERVES 2

PREP TIME: 5 MINUTES • COOK TIME: 8 MINUTES

China's infinitely more delicious and healthful version of chicken fingers.

2 egg whites

¼ cup rice flour

1 red chile, seeded and minced

½ cup finely chopped fresh cilantro

Salt

8 ounces thinly sliced boneless, skinless chicken breast halves (cutlets)

Fresh watercress

Shredded carrots

1 ¾ cups cooked brown rice, warmed

Whisk the egg whites in a shallow bowl. In another bowl, combine the flour, chile, cilantro, and salt to taste. Place the chicken pieces in the egg whites; turn to coat. Dip the chicken in the chile mixture; turn to coat.

Lightly coat a medium nonstick skillet with cooking spray; place over medium heat. Add the chicken; cook for 4 minutes per side, until browned and cooked through.

Arrange the watercress and shredded carrots on a serving platter; top with the chicken. Serve with the rice.

SNACK

Lime-Spiked Peanut Noodles

SERVES 2

PREP TIME: 5 MINUTES • COOK TIME: 5 MINUTES

Peanuts and peanut butter appear in many Chinese dishes. Although these peanut noodles are too high in fat to eat every day, they make a fun and nutritious snack the whole family will love.

TIP: Even though udon (buckwheat) noodles are traditionally a Japanese ingredient we couldn't pass up on their high fiber content here.

3 tablespoons reduced-fat smooth peanut butter

1 clove garlic, smashed

1 tablespoon reduced-sodium soy sauce

1 tablespoon fresh lime juice

2 teaspoons sweet chili sauce

4 ounces udon noodles

½ cup cucumber matchsticks

Lime wedges

In a food processor, pulse the peanut butter, garlic, soy sauce, lime juice, and chili sauce. Add hot water 1 tablespoon at a time until the sauce is the consistency of heavy cream.

Meanwhile, cook the noodles according to the package directions. Drain and rinse in cold water to prevent sticking. Toss with the sauce, garnish with the cucumbers, and serve with lime wedges.

Three-Pea Stir-Fry

SERVES 2

PREP TIME: 5 MINUTES • COOK TIME: 6 MINUTES

Serve this vibrant green dish in the spring, when snow peas are their freshest. If you can't find pea shoots, substitute alfalfa sprouts.

1 teaspoon canola or sesame oil

1 leek, thinly sliced and rinsed clean (white and light green parts only)

4 ounces snow peas, trimmed

½ cup frozen green peas, thawed

1 tablespoon peeled and minced fresh ginger

1 tablespoon reduced-sodium soy sauce

1 tablespoon rice vinegar

1 cup coarsely chopped pea shoots

Salt and black pepper

Warm the oil in a large nonstick skillet over medium-high heat. Add the leek; cook for 2 minutes, stirring. Stir in the snow peas, green peas, ginger, soy sauce, vinegar, and ¼ cup water; sauté for 3 minutes. Add the pea shoots; cook just until wilted, stirring. Season with salt and pepper and serve.

Pork and Cabbage Dumplings

MAKES 18 DUMPLINGS

PREP TIME: 15 MINUTES • COOK TIME: 16 MINUTES

Sure, you can buy premade frozen dumplings, but they are often full of chemicals. It's not hard to make homemade dumplings, which are so much better for you. Although ground pork is a more traditional dumpling filling, a lower-fat option would be ground chicken.

$^3/_4$ cup coleslaw mix

3 ounces lean ground pork or ground chicken breast

2 scallions, thinly sliced

2 teaspoons reduced-sodium soy sauce, plus more for serving

1 teaspoon rice vinegar

$^1/_2$ teaspoon Asian sesame oil

1 egg white, lightly beaten

18 wonton wrappers

In a large bowl, combine the coleslaw, pork, scallions, soy sauce, vinegar, and sesame oil. Fold in the egg white.

Hold a wonton wrapper in your palm. Place 1 rounded teaspoon of filling slightly off-center in the wrapper. Fold one side of the wrapper over the filling. Using your thumb and index finger, seal the wonton by pinching the wrapper together. Moisten the wrapper edges with water to help seal shut.

Coat a large nonstick skillet with cooking spray; place over medium-high heat. Add the wontons; cook for 3 minutes, until golden. Turn the dumplings; cook for 2 minutes. Reduce the heat to low, add $^1/_2$ cup water, and cover. Cook for 8 minutes, until most of the water is absorbed and the wrappers are slightly translucent. Uncover, increase the heat to medium, and cook for 3 minutes, without stirring, until the bottoms are well browned. Transfer to a paper-towel-lined plate to drain. Serve with soy sauce.

Shrimp and Bok Choy Pot Stickers

MAKES 18 POT STICKERS

PREP TIME: 15 MINUTES • COOK TIME: 16 MINUTES

Wonton wrappers, or skins, can be round or square. The method for folding them is the same no matter what the shape.

4 ounces precooked (peeled and deveined) small shrimp, thawed, then
      coarsely chopped

3 ounces baby bok choy, cored and thinly sliced

1 clove garlic, minced

1 teaspoon peeled and minced fresh ginger

2 teaspoons reduced-sodium soy sauce, plus more for serving

1 egg white, lightly beaten

18 wonton wrappers

In a large bowl, combine the shrimp, bok choy, garlic, ginger, and soy sauce. Fold in the egg white.

Hold a wonton wrapper in your palm. Place 1 rounded teaspoon of filling slightly off-center in the wrapper. Fold one side of the wrapper over the filling. Using your thumb and index finger, seal the wonton by pinching the wrapper together. Moisten the wrapper edges with water to help seal shut.

Coat a large nonstick skillet with cooking spray; set over medium-high heat. Add the wontons; cook for 3 minutes, until golden on the bottom. Turn the wontons; cook for 2 minutes. Reduce the heat to low, add ½ cup water, and cover. Cook for 8 minutes, until most of the water is absorbed and the wrappers are slightly translucent. Uncover, increase the heat to medium, and cook for 3 minutes, without stirring, until the bottoms are well browned. Transfer to a paper-towel-lined plate to drain. Serve with soy sauce.

DINNER

Spicy Red-Stewed Salmon with Brown Rice

SERVES 2

PREP TIME: 5 MINUTES • COOK TIME: 10 MINUTES

Red stewing is a method of slow-cooking meat or fish in soy sauce, imparting tons of flavor but no fat.

¼ cup reduced-sodium soy sauce

1 teaspoon Splenda or other sugar substitute

6 scallions, cut into 2-inch pieces

2 cloves garlic, minced

½ red or green chile, seeded

2 salmon fillets (about 4 ounces each)

1½ cups cooked brown rice, warmed

In a deep medium skillet, combine 1 cup water, the soy sauce, Splenda, scallions, garlic, and chile. Bring to a simmer over high heat.

Add the salmon; reduce the heat so that the liquid simmers. Cook for 10 minutes, turning a few times, until cooked through yet still pink inside. Serve on the rice, spooning the cooking sauce over the top. Discard the chile.

Five-Spice Halibut

SERVES 2

PREP TIME: 5 MINUTES (PLUS MARINATING) • COOK TIME: 13 MINUTES

Precooked brown rice is a great way to enjoy fiber-rich rice without the long cooking time. Look for it in the freezer section of health food stores or large supermarkets.

1 teaspoon finely grated lime zest

2 tablespoons fresh lime juice

1 teaspoon olive oil, divided

2 teaspoons peeled and minced fresh ginger

½ teaspoon Chinese five-spice powder

2 halibut fillets (about 5 ounces each)

4 ounces sugar snap peas

2 cloves garlic, sliced

1 ½ cups cooked brown rice, warmed

In a medium nonreactive bowl, combine the lime zest, lime juice, oil, ginger, and five-spice powder. Add the halibut and turn to coat. Refrigerate for 30 minutes or up to 2 hours.

Coat a medium nonstick skillet with cooking spray. Add the fish; cook for 4 minutes per side, until just cooked through. Transfer to a platter; cover to keep warm.

In the same skillet over medium heat, cook the peas for 4 minutes, until tender-crisp, stirring often. Add the garlic; cook for 1 minute. Serve the halibut and peas atop the rice.

Spicy Beef Stir-Fry with Black Bean Sauce

SERVES 2

PREP TIME: 10 MINUTES (PLUS MARINATING) • COOK TIME: 6 MINUTES

Black bean sauce is a salty, bitter blend of fermented black beans and garlic.

8 ounces flank steak, cut into 1-inch cubes

3 tablespoons reduced-sodium soy sauce, divided

3 tablespoons orange juice, divided

2 tablespoons black bean sauce

1 tablespoon sweet chili paste

1 stalk broccoli, cut into small florets, stems thinly sliced

4 ounces bean sprouts

1 ½ cups cooked brown rice, warmed

1 scallion, thinly sliced

In a medium bowl, combine the beef cubes and 2 tablespoons of the soy sauce; marinate for at least 30 minutes.

In a small bowl, whisk the remaining 1 tablespoon soy sauce, the orange juice, black bean sauce, and chili paste.

Coat a large nonstick skillet with cooking spray; set over medium-high heat. Add the broccoli; cook for 2 minutes, stirring. Add ¼ cup water; cover and cook for 1 minute, until crisp-tender. Transfer to a platter.

Lightly coat the skillet again with cooking spray; place over medium heat. Add the marinated beef; cook for 2 minutes, stirring constantly. Add the soy sauce mixture, broccoli, and bean sprouts; cook for 1 minute, until warmed through. Serve over the rice, garnished with the scallions.

Morning Muesli and Hot Coffee

SERVES 2

PREP TIME: 3 MINUTES (PLUS MARINATING)

Weekday mornings find Swedes, like most people, grabbing a quick bowl of cereal and a hot cup of coffee for breakfast. The difference is, instead of a sugar-and-preservative-laden bowl of packaged flakes, many Swedes enjoy a homemade blend of whole oats, nuts, and berries. You may need to add a little more milk or yogurt here to achieve the desired consistency.

TIP: Agave nectar is available at health food and specialty stores. You can also find it at some supermarkets next to the honey.

½ cup old-fashioned or quick-cooking oats

½ cup nonfat plain yogurt

1 cup nonfat milk, divided

1 tablespoon agave nectar

1 teaspoon fresh lemon juice

¼ teaspoon vanilla extract

1 cup fresh blueberries or other berries

3 tablespoons chopped hazelnuts

2 cups hot coffee

In a small bowl, stir the oats, yogurt, ½ cup of the milk, the agave nectar, lemon juice, and vanilla until blended. Cover and refrigerate for at least 1 hour or overnight.

Stir in the remaining ½ cup milk. Top with the berries and nuts. Serve with the coffee.

Swedish Pancakes with Raspberries

SERVES 2

PREP TIME: 5 MINUTES • COOK TIME: 9 MINUTES

The defining aspect of Swedish pancakes is their superthin size. Make these small for a sweet Sunday morning treat. Berries appear often in Swedish food, both fresh, as atop these pancakes, and in sauces for savory dishes.

1 large egg yolk

2 tablespoons Splenda or other sugar substitute

1 teaspoon vanilla extract

Pinch of salt

1 cup nonfat milk

½ cup whole wheat flour

3 tablespoons white flour

3 egg whites

1 cup fresh raspberries

In a medium bowl, whisk the egg yolk, Splenda, vanilla, and salt. Alternately whisk in the milk and flour, stirring well after each addition, to make a thin, smooth batter.

In another bowl, whisk the egg whites until they hold stiff peaks. Gently and quickly fold them into the pancake batter.

Lightly coat a large nonstick skillet with cooking spray; place over medium-high heat. Drop about 2 tablespoons of batter into the skillet for each pancake. Cook as many pancakes at once as will fit comfortably, turning them when they are browned. Total cooking time is about 3 minutes per pancake. Serve with the berries.

Crunchy Toasted Granola

SERVES 2: MAKES 2 CUPS

PREP TIME: 2 MINUTES • COOK TIME: 25 MINUTES

Since this crunchy, satisfying, fiber-rich cereal is relatively high in fat and calories, serve it only on special occasions.

TIP: Keep an eye on the cereal as it bakes—it burns quickly!

2 cups old-fashioned or quick-cooking oats

2 tablespoons chopped natural almonds

½ teaspoon ground cinnamon

Pinch of salt

2 tablespoons agave nectar

2 tablespoons chopped dried apricots

Nonfat milk

Preheat the oven to 325°F. In a large bowl, combine the oats, almonds, cinnamon, and salt. In a small cup, heat the agave nectar in the microwave just until warm. Fold it into the oat mixture, stirring to coat well.

Spread the cereal on a large rimmed baking sheet. Bake for 20 to 25 minutes, stirring often to prevent burning. Rotate the pan after stirring. The cereal is done when it seems mostly dry and no longer sticky. Let cool for 15 minutes on the baking sheet. Transfer to a medium bowl. Divide into 2 serving bowls; serve with the apricots and milk as desired.

LUNCH

Oven-Baked Swedish Meatballs

SERVES 2

PREP TIME: 10 MINUTES • COOK TIME: 15 MINUTES

Spaghetti and meatballs—Swedish style!

8 ounces extra-lean ground beef

½ small onion, minced

1 egg white

¼ teaspoon Worcestershire sauce

Salt and black pepper

Pinch of ground cinnamon

Pinch of ground cardamom

Pinch of ground allspice

4 ounces whole wheat egg noodles or pasta

Preheat the oven to 375°F. In a large bowl, combine all the ingredients except the noodles. Using your hands, form small balls. Arrange in a large roasting pan—make sure the meatballs aren't touching—and bake for 15 minutes, turning occasionally to cook on all sides.

Meanwhile, cook the noodles according to the package directions. Drain.

Serve the meatballs atop the noodles.

Creamed Herring on Brown Bread

SERVES 2

PREP TIME: 3 MINUTES

Look for pickled herring in the refrigerated section of gourmet food shops. It is rich in heart-healthy omega-3 fatty acids, so the fat content is higher than for many other types of seafood.

    2 thin slices brown or dark rye bread, toasted
    2 tablespoons nonfat sour cream
    3 ounces pickled herring, drained
    1 cup alfalfa sprouts or chopped romaine lettuce
    2 tablespoons fresh lemon juice

Spread the toast evenly with sour cream. Arrange the herring, then the sprouts on top. Drizzle evenly with the lemon juice and serve immediately.

SNACK

Creamy Apple, Celery, and Red Onion Salad

SERVES 2

PREP TIME: 5 MINUTES

The growing season is short in Scandinavia, so salads are often composed of fruits and vegetables that will keep for a long time, such as apples and onions.

1½ Granny Smith or Golden Delicious apples, cored and thinly sliced

2 stalks celery, very thinly sliced

2 tablespoons chopped red onion

½ cup nonfat sour cream

½ cup nonfat plain Greek yogurt

2 tablespoons minced fresh dill

1 teaspoon rice vinegar

Pinch of salt

Boston lettuce, watercress, or baby spinach

2 slices rye bread, toasted

In a medium bowl, combine the apples, celery, onion, sour cream, yogurt, dill, vinegar, and salt; toss to combine. Refrigerate for at least 20 minutes. Arrange the lettuce on a platter; top with the salad. Serve with the toast.

Golden Split Pea Soup

SERVES 2

PREP TIME: 5 MINUTES • COOK TIME: 45 MINUTES

Traditionally eaten on Thursday, Scandinavian pea soup is often served with a pot of mustard for diners to swirl into their bowls. Swedish pancakes, with jam or berries (see recipe page 167), are a popular accompaniment. Since this is a snack, serve with toast points.

½ teaspoon olive oil

2 carrots, chopped

1 small onion, chopped

1 stalk celery, chopped

Salt and black pepper

1 cup yellow or green split peas

½ ham hock, well rinsed

1 teaspoon chopped fresh thyme

3 cups vegetable or reduced-sodium chicken broth

2 slices rye or whole-grain bread, toasted and cut into triangles

Warm the oil in a medium saucepan over medium-low heat. Add the carrots, onion, celery, and salt and pepper to taste. Cook for 4 minutes, stirring often. Add the split peas, ham hock, thyme, and broth. Bring to a simmer; reduce the heat to low and cook for 40 minutes, stirring often and adding up to 1 cup water to maintain a soupy consistency.

Transfer about half of the soup to a blender; purée. (Alternatively, purée in the pot with an immersion blender after removing the ham hock.) Remove the ham hock; chop about ¼ cup meat from the bone. Discard the bone.

Return the puréed soup and chopped ham to the pot; warm through. Season with salt and pepper. Serve with the toast points.

Smoked Trout and Horseradish Cream Open-Faced Sandwich

SERVES 2

PREP TIME: 5 MINUTES

The Swedes are known for their smoked and cured fish. Smoked trout can be found at gourmet stores or in the canned fish aisle of large supermarkets.

2 tablespoons nonfat sour cream

2 teaspoons horseradish sauce

2 slices rye or whole-grain bread, toasted

2 ounces skinless smoked trout fillet

1 pear, cored and thinly sliced

$\frac{1}{2}$ cup baby arugula or baby spinach

In a small cup, combine the sour cream and horseradish sauce. Spread half the cream on the toast. Top with the trout and pear slices. Arrange the arugula on top and serve.

Pickled Cucumber
with Fresh Dill on Rye Crisps

SERVES 2

PREP TIME: 5 MINUTES

English cucumbers are relatively seedless, which is preferred here.

TIP: To seed a cucumber, cut in half lengthwise, then run the tip of a teaspoon along the channel of seeds, scraping out the seeds as you go.

1 cucumber or ½ English cucumber, unpeeled and very thinly sliced

1 tablespoon white vinegar

2 tablespoons chopped fresh dill

1 tablespoon minced red onion

Salt

¼ teaspoon Splenda or other sugar substitute

4 large rye crisp crackers

1 cup nonfat cottage cheese

In a small bowl or plastic container, combine all the ingredients except the crackers and cottage cheese. Cover and refrigerate for at least 3 hours. Top each cracker with ½ cup of cottage cheese and some cucumber salad; serve.

Blueberry Rye Muffins

MAKES 12 MUFFINS

PREP TIME: 10 MINUTES • COOK TIME: 16 MINUTES

Baking is an important part of the Scandinavian culture. These muffins could be served for breakfast, as a snack, or with dinner.

TIP: Flaxseeds are rich in omega-3 fatty acids, which have been found to help lower cholesterol. The seeds must be ground for the body to absorb their nutrients. Use a spice or coffee grinder to grind them.

1 cup dark rye flour

1 cup whole wheat flour or whole wheat pastry flour

¼ cup ground flaxseeds

1 teaspoon salt

1 teaspoon baking powder

½ teaspoon baking soda

1 cup nonfat milk

3 egg whites

¼ cup canola oil

3 tablespoons agave nectar

1 cup frozen blueberries or raspberries

¾ cup nonfat plain yogurt for each serving

Preheat the oven to 400°F. Line a muffin tin with paper liners.

In a large mixing bowl, combine the flours, flaxseeds, salt, baking powder, and baking soda. In another bowl, whisk the milk, egg whites, oil, and agave nectar. Fold the liquid ingredients into the dry ingredients until just blended. Fold in the berries.

Drop the batter into the lined muffin cups. Bake for 16 minutes, until a toothpick inserted in the center comes out clean. Transfer to a wire rack to cool. Serve with the yogurt.

Smoked Salmon Smorgasbord

SERVES 2

PREP TIME: 5 MINUTES

Smoked salmon is an everyday, year-round staple in Swedish households. Because of its strong flavor, only a small amount is needed.

   1 teaspoon honey mustard or Dijon mustard

   1 teaspoon fresh lemon juice

   1 teaspoon canola oil

   2 tablespoons chopped fresh dill

   4 rusks or rye crisp crackers

   4 slices smoked salmon (about 3 ounces total)

   1 apple, cored and thinly sliced

In a small bowl, whisk the mustard and lemon juice to blend. Gradually whisk in the oil. Stir in the dill.

Arrange the crackers on a platter; top with the salmon and sauce. Serve with the apple slices.

DINNER

Poached Salmon with Herbed Mayonnaise

SERVES 2

PREP TIME: 5 MINUTES • COOK TIME: 13 MINUTES

Poaching is a great cooking method, as it imparts a delicate flavor and a moist texture to foods without adding any fat. This heart-healthy salmon is served with a fresh-herb-flecked creamy sauce, warm bulgur, and a tossed green salad.

½ cup bulgur

Sauce

2 tablespoons nonfat mayonnaise

2 teaspoons fresh lemon juice

2 tablespoons chopped fresh tarragon

2 tablespoons chopped fresh flat-leaf parsley

1 tablespoon chopped fresh chives

Salt and black pepper

Salmon

1 cup dry white wine

2 salmon fillets (about 4 ounces each)

Salt and black pepper

Tossed Salad (see page 178)

Cook the bulgur according to the package directions.

To make the sauce, in a small cup, combine the mayonnaise and lemon juice. Add the herbs and stir until combined. Season with salt and pepper. Refrigerate until serving.

To cook the salmon, in a deep medium skillet, bring the wine and 2 cups water to a simmer over high heat. Season the salmon with salt and pepper. Submerge the fillets, skin side down, in the simmering liquid. Add hot water if necessary to just cover the salmon. Cover and poach at a bare simmer for 8 minutes, until just cooked through. Let cool for

5 minutes in the cooking water. Serve at room temperature or chilled with the sauce, bulgur, and salad. You can serve the sauce on top or on the side.

Tossed Salad: In a medium bowl, toss 2 cups chopped romaine lettuce and 1 cup chopped tomatoes. Squeeze a lemon wedge over the salad.

Roasted Pork Tenderloin with Apples

SERVES 2

PREP TIME: 5 MINUTES • COOK TIME: 23 MINUTES

Pork tenderloin is a lean, quick-cooking cut of meat. Here it's roasted with apples and served with warm barley.

1 small pork tenderloin (about 8 ounces), trimmed

Salt and black pepper

2 teaspoons chopped fresh thyme

1 teaspoon olive oil

2 green apples, each cut crosswise, or horizontally, into 3 rounds

½ cup barley

½ cup white wine or apple cider

Preheat the oven to 400°F. Pat the pork dry with a paper towel. Season with salt and pepper and sprinkle with the thyme.

Warm the oil in a large ovenproof skillet over medium-high heat. Sear the pork until browned on all sides, about 8 minutes. In the last 2 minutes of cooking, add the apples, cut side down.

Turn the apples over and transfer the skillet to the oven. Roast for 12 minutes, until the internal temperature of the pork reaches 145°F for medium.

Meanwhile, cook the barley according to the package directions. Keep warm.

Transfer the pork to a cutting board; tent with aluminum foil to keep warm. Remove the apples to a serving platter.

Place the skillet over medium-high heat. Add the wine; cook for 3 minutes, until the wine is reduced by half.

Slice the meat and transfer to the platter with the apples; add cooked barley. Drizzle the pan sauce over the pork and barley; serve.

Whole Wheat Crêpes with Fresh Raspberries

SERVES 2

PREP TIME: 5 MINUTES • COOK TIME: 5 MINUTES

Crêpes are considered a national dish of France. They are incredibly versatile, as they can be served with berries for breakfast or filled with meat or cheese for lunch or dinner.

½ cup whole wheat pastry flour or whole wheat flour

½ teaspoon baking powder

¼ teaspoon salt

1 whole egg

1 egg white

5 ounces nonfat milk (about ⅔ cup)

¼ teaspoon vanilla extract

1 ½ cups nonfat plain yogurt

1 ½ cups fresh raspberries

In a medium bowl, whisk the flour, baking powder, and salt.

In another bowl, whisk the whole egg and egg white. Whisk in the milk and vanilla until blended.

Lightly coat an 8-inch nonstick skillet with cooking spray; place over medium heat. Pour in about ⅓ cup batter, tilting and rotating the skillet to coat the bottom. Cook for 10 seconds, until just set and pale golden around the edge. Run a rubber spatula around the edge of the crêpe to loosen it. Using your fingers, carefully flip it over. Cook for 20 seconds, until the underside is set. Transfer to a plate.

Repeat with the remaining batter to make 3 more crêpes. Serve with the yogurt and raspberries.

Asparagus Mini-Soufflés with Chives

SERVES 1

PREP TIME: 5 MINUTES • COOK TIME: 32 MINUTES

Serve these light and elegant soufflés in small porcelain ramekins. Each ramekin should hold 8 ounces. If you don't own any ramekins, you can use ovenproof custard cups instead. This recipe is easily doubled to serve 2.

TIP: The easiest way to cut fresh chives is to snip them with scissors.

4 asparagus spears, cut into 1-inch pieces

1 whole egg

2 egg whites

2 tablespoons nonfat half-and-half or nonfat plain yogurt

Salt and black pepper to taste

2 tablespoons minced fresh chives

2 tablespoons shredded Parmesan or Gruyère cheese, divided

2 slices whole-grain bread

Preheat the oven to 350°F. Lightly coat two 8-ounce ramekins with cooking spray.

Lightly coat a medium nonstick skillet with cooking spray; place over medium heat. Add the asparagus; cook for 2 minutes, until slightly charred, shaking the pan occasionally.

In a medium bowl, whisk the whole egg, egg whites, half-and-half, salt and pepper, chives, and 1 tablespoon of the cheese. Stir in the asparagus.

Place the ramekins on a rimmed baking sheet. Ladle the egg mixture into the ramekins; sprinkle with the remaining 1 tablespoon cheese. Bake for 30 minutes, until puffed up but slightly firm. Remove from the oven and serve with bread. The soufflés may fall upon cooling.

Note: For the quickest French-style breakfast ever, spread a little sugar-free fruit preserves on a thin slice of whole-grain toast. Serve with café au lait—equal parts hot nonfat milk and coffee.

Easy Niçoise Salad

SERVES 2

PREP TIME: 10 MINUTES • COOK TIME: 3 MINUTES

The French call this a *salade composé,* which means the ingredients are arranged on a platter and drizzled with dressing, rather than being tossed.

4 ounces green beans, trimmed and cut in half

1 can (6 ounces) solid albacore tuna packed in water, drained and
    squeezed dry

4 tablespoons light red wine vinegar dressing, divided

Salt

4 cups baby lettuce

1 medium tomato, cored and thinly sliced

2 hard-boiled eggs

4 thin slices whole-grain baguette

Bring a small saucepan of water to a boil over high heat. Add the beans; cook for 3 minutes, until crisp-tender. Drain and rinse with cool water.

In a small bowl, mix the tuna and 2 tablespoons of the dressing until combined. Season with salt.

On a medium platter, arrange the lettuce, tomato slices, beans, and tuna. Drizzle with the remaining 2 tablespoons dressing. Remove and discard the egg yolks. Slice the egg whites and arrange on the platter. Serve with the baguette.

Warm Lentils with Goat Cheese

SERVES 2

PREP TIME: 5 MINUTES • COOK TIME: 35 MINUTES

Dried beans and lentils are a household staple in southern France. This homey, hearty dish can serve as a side with dinner or as a luncheon main course.

Lentils

³⁄₄ cup dried green lentils, washed and picked over

1 shallot, cut in half

Salt

Dressing

1 tablespoon sherry vinegar or red wine vinegar

1 clove garlic, minced

1 teaspoon Dijon mustard

1 teaspoon olive oil

Salt and black pepper

¼ cup chopped fresh flat-leaf parsley

2 ounces reduced-fat goat cheese, cut into rounds

To cook the lentils, in a medium saucepan combine the lentils, shallot, and salt. Add enough water to cover by 1½ inches. Bring to a simmer; cover and cook for 15 minutes, until the lentils are tender all the way through but not mushy. Set a strainer over a bowl and drain.

Discard the shallot. Return the cooking liquid to the pot and bring to a boil. Simmer for 10 minutes to reduce the liquid and concentrate the flavors.

Preheat the oven to 350°F.

To make the dressing, in a medium bowl whisk ¼ cup of the lentil cooking liquid, the vinegar, garlic, mustard, and oil. Season with salt and pepper. Add the cooked lentils; toss to coat. Stir in the parsley. Spoon into a pie plate or small casserole dish; top with the goat cheese rounds. Bake for 10 minutes, until the cheese is softened and the dish is warmed through. Serve.

Soupe au Pistou

SERVES 2

PREP TIME: 10 MINUTES • COOK TIME: 28 MINUTES

Originally, *pistou* was the French name for a basil-garlic purée, much like the Italians' pesto. It is also the name of a simple vegetable soup that's garnished with basil.

TIP: The French love to use leeks in their cooking. If leeks are unavailable in your market, substitute yellow onion.

1 teaspoon olive oil

1 cup sliced leek (about 1/2 leek), rinsed clean (white and light green parts only)

1 carrot, thinly sliced

2 cloves garlic, minced

1 cup canned diced tomatoes, with liquid

1 ½ cups reduced-sodium chicken broth

½ small zucchini, diced

½ teaspoon *herbes de Provence* or dried thyme

Salt and black pepper to taste

1 cup canned white kidney or cannellini beans, drained and rinsed

3 ounces green beans, trimmed and cut into 1-inch lengths

¼ cup slivered fresh basil leaves, or ¼ cup basil purée

2 tablespoons grated Parmesan cheese

Warm the oil in a medium saucepan over medium-low heat. Add the leeks and carrot; cook for 4 minutes, until softened, stirring often. Add the garlic; cook for 1 minute, stirring. Stir in the tomatoes; cook for 8 minutes, stirring often. Stir in the broth, zucchini, *herbes de Provence,* and salt and pepper; bring to a simmer. Reduce the heat to low, cover, and simmer for 10 minutes. Stir in the canned beans and green beans. Simmer for 5 minutes, until the green beans are crisp-tender and the soup is warmed through. Transfer to 2 bowls; garnish with the basil and Parmesan.

THE 5-FACTOR WORLD DIET RECIPES   185

Open-Faced Chicken and
Caramelized Onion Sandwich

SERVES 2

PREP TIME: 2 MINUTES • COOK TIME: 27 MINUTES

Thinly sliced boneless, skinless chicken breasts, sometimes called cutlets, cook in minutes. Substitute half of a precooked chicken breast if
you like.

TIP: Cooking sliced onions at a low heat for a long time caramelizes
their natural sugars and lends a sweetness to them.

1 large onion, cut in half and very thinly sliced (about 3 cups)

1 tablespoon balsamic vinegar

Salt and black pepper to taste

2 thinly sliced boneless, skinless chicken breast halves (cutlets; about
   2 ½ ounces each)

1 small whole-grain baguette (about 8 inches), cut in half horizontally

Coat a large nonstick skillet with nonstick cooking spray; place over
medium-low heat. Add the onion; cook for 15 minutes, stirring often.
Add up to 2 tablespoons water and reduce the heat if the onion begins
to scorch. Add the vinegar, and salt and pepper to taste; cook for 4 minutes, until golden, stirring often. Scrape the onions onto a plate.

Coat the skillet again with cooking spray; place over medium heat.
Season the chicken with salt and pepper. Add to the skillet and cook for
4 minutes per side, until cooked through.

Meanwhile, toast the baguette halves. Top each half with a chicken
cutlet and some onion. Serve.

Balsamic Roasted Tomato and Goat Cheese Crisps

SERVES 2

PREP TIME: 5 MINUTES • COOK TIME: 10 MINUTES

The French like to cook using small amounts of intensely flavored ingredients, such as balsamic vinegar and goat cheese.

8 cherry tomatoes

2 teaspoons balsamic vinegar

Salt and black pepper

¼ cup canned white kidney or cannellini beans, drained and rinsed

½ teaspoon olive oil

4 large whole-grain crisp crackers

1 ounce reduced-fat goat cheese, crumbled

8 baby arugula leaves

Preheat the oven to 350°F. In an 8-inch square baking dish, toss the tomatoes with the vinegar and salt and pepper to taste until coated. Bake for 8 to 10 minutes, until the tomatoes are soft, shaking the pan occasionally.

In a small bowl, mash the beans and oil to form a thick paste.

Top each cracker with white bean paste, 2 warm tomatoes, a sprinkling of cheese, and 2 arugula leaves. Serve.

Warm Ratatouille

SERVES 2

PREP TIME: 10 MINUTES • COOK TIME: 8 MINUTES

This classic Provençal side dish can be served on its own or as a dip, pasta sauce, pizza topping, or sandwich filling. For a quick snack, serve with whole-grain bread for scooping.

½ eggplant, diced

½ zucchini, diced

1 red bell pepper, diced

½ shallot, minced, or ¼ cup finely chopped red onion

1 clove garlic, chopped

1-2 cups canned diced tomatoes with basil

½ cup canned white kidney or cannellini beans, drained and rinsed

3 tablespoons chopped fresh basil

2 tablespoons grated Parmesan cheese

Lightly coat a medium nonstick skillet with cooking spray; place over medium heat. Add the eggplant; cook for 4 minutes, stirring. Add the zucchini, pepper, shallot, garlic, 1 cup of the tomatoes, and the beans; cook for 4 minutes, stirring. Stir in up to 1 more cup tomatoes to create the desired consistency.

Spoon the ratatouille into 2 serving bowls. Top each serving with half the basil and cheese.

Roasted Asparagus with Quinoa and Parmesan Curls

SERVES 2

PREP TIME: 3 MINUTES • COOK TIME: 10 MINUTES

Though not part of classic French cooking, quinoa is now a hugely popular grain in the country. Since it's one of those miracle foods that contain both fiber and protein, its popularity is well deserved.

TIP: This dish is especially good when made in the spring, when asparagus is at its best.

½ cup quinoa

Salt

Black pepper

10 asparagus spears, preferably thin

½ shallot, minced

1 tablespoon fresh lemon juice

½ teaspoon olive oil

1 ounce Parmesan cheese, shaved into curls

In a small saucepan, bring ¾ cup water to a boil over high heat. Add the quinoa and a pinch of salt; bring back to a boil. Reduce the heat to low; cover and simmer for about 6 minutes, until nearly all of the water has been absorbed and the quinoa is tender but not soft.

Meanwhile, preheat the oven to 400°F. In a 9-by-13-inch baking dish, toss the asparagus with the shallot, lemon juice, oil, and salt and pepper to taste until coated. Roast for 8 to 10 minutes, shaking the dish three times.

Preheat the broiler. Top the asparagus with the cheese; broil for 30 seconds. Serve atop the quinoa.

DINNER

Lemon-Caper Braised Halibut

SERVES 2

PREP TIME: 5 MINUTES • COOK TIME: 11 MINUTES

TIP: Capers are sold pickled in a vinegary brine. They should be drained and rinsed before using.

2 halibut fillets (about 5 ounces each)

Salt and black pepper

1 teaspoon olive oil

1 ½ cups cherry tomatoes cut in half

2 tablespoons capers, drained and rinsed

2 tablespoons fresh lemon juice

4 cups baby spinach

2 tablespoons chopped fresh flat-leaf parsley

2 slices whole-grain bread or 2 chunks whole-grain baguette

Season the halibut with salt and pepper. Coat a medium nonstick skillet with cooking spray; place over medium-high heat. Add the fish; cook for 5 minutes per side, until cooked through. Transfer to a platter and cover to keep warm.

Reduce the heat to low. Add the oil, tomatoes, capers, and lemon juice; cook for 1 minute, stirring. Arrange the spinach on 2 serving plates; top with the fish. Spoon the sauce over the halibut and garnish with the parsley. Serve with the bread.

Moules Marinades

SERVES 2

PREP TIME: 10 MINUTES • COOK TIME: 15 MINUTES

This classic Mediterranean dish depends on the freshest ingredients. Always select tightly closed mussels: this means they are still alive.

1¼ pounds fresh mussels

1 teaspoon olive oil

3 shallots, coarsely chopped

4 cloves garlic, coarsely chopped

1 cup dry white wine

4 plum tomatoes, chopped, or 4 canned plum tomatoes, drained

¼ cup chopped fresh flat-leaf parsley

2 slices whole-grain baguette

Thoroughly rinse and scrub the mussels; rinse with several changes of water. Discard any mussels that are open.

Warm the oil in a medium saucepan over medium heat. Add the shallots and garlic; cook for 3 minutes, stirring. Add the mussels and wine; cover and cook for 5 minutes, until all the mussels open. Using a slotted spoon, remove the mussels from the pan and put in a bowl. Discard any that have not opened. Strain the cooking liquid through a colander; reserve.

Using a paper towel, wipe out the saucepan; return the strained liquid to the pan. Add the tomatoes; bring to a boil over high heat. Cook for 4 minutes, stirring to incorporate the flavors and smashing the tomatoes.

Transfer the mussels to 2 serving bowls. Spoon the tomato sauce over the mussels and garnish with the parsley. Serve with the baguette.

Garlic Chicken Cassoulet

SERVES 2

PREP TIME: 12 MINUTES (PLUS MARINADE) • COOK TIME: 30 MINUTES

TIP: The easiest way to clean leeks? Slice them, then place the slices in a colander and rinse thoroughly, using your fingers to separate the rings and dislodge the grit.

3 cloves garlic, minced and divided

2 teaspoons chopped fresh rosemary, or 1 teaspoon dried

1 teaspoon chopped fresh thyme, or $\frac{1}{2}$ teaspoon dried

1 tablespoon balsamic vinegar

2 boneless, skinless chicken breast halves (about 4 ounces each)

2 carrots, thickly sliced

1 leek, thinly sliced and rinsed clean (white and light green parts only)

Salt and black pepper

1 cup canned white kidney or cannellini beans, rinsed and drained, $\frac{1}{4}$ cup liquid reserved

In a medium nonreactive bowl, combine half the garlic, the rosemary, thyme, and vinegar. Add the chicken; turn to coat. Cover and refrigerate for at least 30 minutes or up to 2 hours.

Preheat the oven to 375°F. Lightly coat a deep medium nonstick skillet with cooking spray; place over medium heat. Add the chicken; cook for 2 minutes per side, until golden brown but not cooked through. Transfer to a platter.

In the same skillet, cook the carrots, leek, and remaining garlic for 5 minutes, stirring to scrape up the browned bits from the chicken. Season with salt and pepper. Add the beans, reserved liquid, and 1 cup water. Bring to a simmer; cook for 5 minutes, stirring often. The mixture should be stewlike; add water if it seems too dry.

Nestle the chicken atop the beans. Transfer the skillet to the oven; bake for 12 minutes, until the chicken is cooked through. Serve.

Italian Frittata with Zucchini, Leeks, and Parmesan

SERVES 2

PREP TIME: 5 MINUTES • COOK TIME: 17 MINUTES

The beauty of a frittata, a traditional Italian egg pie, is that it can be served warm or at room temperature for any meal.

TIP: Asiago is a hard grating cheese, similar to Parmesan.

2 leeks, thinly sliced and rinsed clean (white and light green parts only)

1 small zucchini, diced

Salt and black pepper

5 egg whites

½ cup chopped fresh basil

¼ cup grated Parmesan or Asiago cheese

4 slices medium whole-grain baguette, toasted

Preheat the oven to 350°F. Lightly coat a medium ovenproof nonstick skillet with cooking spray; place over medium heat. Add the leeks and zucchini and season with salt and pepper. Cook for 5 minutes, until softened, stirring. Transfer to a bowl.

In another bowl, beat the egg whites until well blended. Whisk in salt and pepper to taste.

Using a paper towel, wipe out the skillet. Lightly coat it with cooking spray and place over medium heat. Add the egg whites; top with the leek mixture, basil, and cheese. Cook for 2 minutes without stirring. Transfer to the oven; bake for 8 to 10 minutes, until just set. Cut into wedges and serve directly out of the skillet while warm, accompanied by the baguette.

Orange-Almond Biscotti with Caffè Latte

SERVES 4

PREP TIME: 5 MINUTES • COOK TIME: 38 MINUTES

Italians love sweets in the morning. The healthy difference is that they eat only a small amount, such as these crispy, nutty cookies. They are delicious dunked in creamy yogurt or your morning latte.

TIP: The cookies will keep for at least a week, tightly covered.

¼ cup whole almonds

¼ cup Splenda or other sugar substitute

2 teaspoons olive oil

1 tablespoon orange juice

2 egg whites

1 egg yolk

¾ cup plus 1 tablespoon whole wheat flour

1 teaspoon baking powder

Pinch of salt

¼ teaspoon orange extract

1 teaspoon grated orange zest

2 cups nonfat plain or vanilla yogurt

2 cups Caffé Latte

Preheat the oven to 350°F. Place the almonds on a rimmed baking sheet and toast for 5 minutes; coarsely chop. Keep the oven at 350°F.

In a small bowl, whisk the Splenda, oil, and orange juice. Beat in the egg whites and egg yolk.

In a separate bowl, whisk together the flour, baking powder, and salt. Gradually add the flour mixture to the egg mixture. Add the orange extract, orange zest, and chopped almonds. Mix until the dough clings together; do not overmix.

Line a baking sheet with parchment paper. Drop the batter onto the sheet, then use your hands to form it into a rounded log about 7 inches by 2 inches. Bake for 25 minutes, until golden brown. Remove from the oven; carefully transfer to a cutting board.

Using a sharp or serrated knife, slice into ½-inch diagonal slices while still warm. Place the slices back on the baking sheet, standing them up on the flat bottoms. Bake for 8 minutes, until firm to the touch. Let cool completely.

Serve the cookies with yogurt for dipping and the coffee.

Nonfat Latte: Steam 1 cup nonfat milk in cappuccino maker, microwave, or small saucepan. Add 2 shots hot espresso. Pour into 2 demitasse cups.

LUNCH

Whole Wheat Pasta with Basil and Spinach Pesto

SERVES 2

PREP TIME: 5 MINUTES • COOK TIME: 10 MINUTES

This recipe makes twice as much pesto as you'll need for the pasta. Set aside half of the sauce (before adding water) and refrigerate for future quick pasta dinners. It also works as a spread for sandwiches or home-made pizza.

Pesto

1 cup packed spinach leaves

2 cups fresh basil leaves

¼ cup canned white kidney or cannellini beans

1 clove garlic, smashed

1 teaspoon extra-virgin olive oil

2 tablespoons grated Parmesan cheese

2 tablespoons pine nuts or walnuts

Pasta

4 ounces whole wheat penne or other tube pasta

Salt and black pepper

2 ounces Parmesan cheese, grated

To make the pesto, in a food processor combine the spinach, basil, beans, garlic, and oil. Process until smooth. Add the cheese and nuts; process until well blended. Transfer half of the sauce to a covered resealable container (not metal) and refrigerate. Place the remaining sauce in a medium serving bowl.

In medium saucepan, cook the pasta according to the package directions. Remove ¼ cup cooking water and stir into the pesto. Drain the pasta. Toss the warm pasta with the pesto and salt and pepper to taste. Garnish with the cheese and serve.

Pan Bagna

SERVES 2

PREP TIME: 5 MINUTES

Although most Italians would probably use tuna packed in olive oil, the water-packed variety lends the same flavor without the added fat.

1 small whole-grain baguette (about 8 inches long)

1 can (6 ounces) solid albacore tuna packed in water, drained and
   squeezed dry

1 tomato, seeded and chopped

3 tablespoons light balsamic dressing

1 tablespoon capers, drained and rinsed

Salt and black pepper

1 ½ cups baby arugula or watercress leaves

Cut the baguette in half horizontally. Scoop out the soft inner bread from both halves, leaving ½-inch-thick shells. Reserve ½ cup bread crumbs.

In a medium bowl, combine the bread crumbs, tuna, tomato, dressing, capers, and salt and pepper to taste. Spoon the mixture into the bottom bread shell. Add the arugula and replace the top of the baguette. Cut crosswise and serve.

Sweet Potato Risotto with Veal Cutlets

SERVES 2

PREP TIME: 10 MINUTES • COOK TIME: 45 MINUTES

Risotto is traditionally made by slowly adding simmering broth to rice as it cooks. Here the method is streamlined, but the result is still a creamy, satisfying pot of rice.

> 2 tablespoons finely chopped red onion
>
> ½ cup brown rice
>
> 1 can (14½ ounces) reduced-sodium chicken broth, divided
>
> 1 small sweet potato (about 7 ounces), peeled and cut into small dice
>
> 2 tablespoons nonfat half-and-half
>
> ½ teaspoon minced fresh sage leaves, or a pinch of dried sage
>
> Salt and black pepper
>
> 2 thinly sliced veal cutlets (about 3 ounces each), pounded to about ¼ inch thick
>
> 3 tablespoons grated Parmesan cheese

Lightly coat a medium nonstick saucepan with cooking spray; place over medium-low heat. Add the onion; cook for 2 minutes, until softened, stirring often. Add the rice; stir to coat. Add 1½ cups of the broth; bring to a simmer. Reduce the heat to very low, cover, and cook for 35 to 40 minutes, until the broth is absorbed and the rice is tender.

Meanwhile, bring a small pot of water to a boil. Add the sweet potato; cook for 10 minutes, until just tender. Drain.

Add the sweet potato, remaining broth, and ½ cup water to the rice, still over low heat. Stir slowly for about 5 minutes, until the broth is incorporated. Stir in the half-and-half and sage. Keep stirring, adding water if necessary, until the rice has the desired consistency. Season with salt and pepper.

Coat a medium nonstick skillet with cooking spray; place over medium-high heat. Season the veal with salt and pepper. Add to the hot pan; cook for 2 minutes per side, until just cooked through. Arrange the veal and risotto on 2 serving plates, sprinkling the cheese over the rice. Serve.

SNACK

Crostini Caprese

SERVES 2

PREP TIME: 5 MINUTES • COOK TIME: 5 MINUTES

These delicious bites are a fun take on the classic tomato, basil, and mozzarella salad. You can substitute any thin whole-grain bread for the crackers.

6 large whole-grain crisp crackers

1 tomato, cored and thinly sliced

2 ounces (½ cup) shredded fat-free mozzarella cheese

½ teaspoon extra virgin olive oil

2 teaspoons balsamic vinegar

1 cup small fresh basil leaves

Salt and black pepper

Preheat the oven to 250°F. Arrange the crackers on a baking sheet. Top with the tomato slices, and sprinkle with cheese. Bake for 5 minutes, until the cheese melts.

Drizzle the crostini with the oil and vinegar. Garnish with the basil leaves and season with salt and pepper. Serve.

Charred Sweet Peppers with Ricotta

SERVES 2

PREP TIME: 10 MINUTES   •   COOK TIME: 10 MINUTES

Roasted red peppers appear in many Italian dishes. Here the peppers are simply tossed with creamy ricotta cheese and fresh basil.

TIP: Use the flame of your gas stove to char the peppers. If you don't have a gas stove, use your grill or broiler.

2 red, orange, or yellow bell peppers

1 teaspoon white or red wine vinegar

Salt and black pepper

⅓ cup part-skim ricotta cheese

¼ cup chopped fresh basil or flat-leaf parsley

2 slices whole-grain baguette

Using tongs, hold 1 bell pepper directly over the flame of your gas stove. When the skin on one side is charred, give the pepper a quarter turn. Continue turning until the whole pepper is charred. Repeat with the other pepper. (Or place both on the grill and follow the same procedure.) Place the peppers in a medium bowl and cover. Let cool for 10 minutes.

Hold 1 roasted pepper over another bowl. Make a slit in the bottom and squeeze to collect the juices in the bowl. Repeat with the other pepper. Cut the peppers in half, then remove and discard the seeds and stem. Using a dull knife or your fingers, rub the charred skin off the peppers, then cut the peppers into strips or cubes.

Whisk the pepper juices, vinegar, and salt and pepper to taste. Add the peppers, ricotta, and basil; toss to coat. Serve with the baguette.

Stuffed Portobello Mushrooms

SERVES 2

PREP TIME: 10 MINUTES • COOK TIME: 25 MINUTES

2 portobello mushrooms

1 teaspoon olive oil

1 teaspoon balsamic vinegar

Salt and black pepper

1 leek, thinly sliced and rinsed clean (white and light green parts only)

2 cups spinach leaves

½ cup canned white kidney or cannellini beans, drained and rinsed

2 tablespoons grated Parmesan cheese

Preheat the oven to 450°F. Set the mushrooms gill side up on a rimmed baking sheet. Drizzle with the oil and vinegar and season with salt and pepper. Bake for 15 minutes.

Meanwhile, coat a large nonstick skillet with cooking spray; place over medium heat. Add the leek; cook for 5 minutes, stirring. Add the spinach a handful at a time, stirring constantly, until it cooks down. Stir in the beans and salt and pepper to taste; cook for 1 minute to combine the flavors.

Fill the mushroom cavities with the spinach mixture. Sprinkle with the cheese. Bake for 10 minutes, until the mushrooms are warmed through and the cheese is melted. Serve.

Eggplant Caponata

MAKES 2 CUPS

PREP TIME: 5 MINUTES • COOK TIME: 18 MINUTES

This classic Sicilian relish is endlessly adaptable. Use it as a pasta sauce or pizza topping. Or serve simply with warm bread.

1 teaspoon olive oil

½ eggplant, cut into small cubes

1 bell pepper (any color), diced

½ onion, diced

1 stalk celery, thinly sliced

¾ cup tomato juice or V8

¼ cup canned lentils, drained and rinsed

1 tablespoon red wine vinegar

2 teaspoons capers, drained and rinsed

Salt and black pepper

3 tablespoons grated Parmesan cheese

Warm the oil in a large skillet over medium heat. Add the eggplant; cook for 4 minutes, until softened, stirring often. Transfer to a bowl.

Lightly coat the skillet again with cooking spray; place over medium heat. Add the bell pepper, onion, and celery; cook for 3 minutes, stirring often.

Add the eggplant, tomato juice, and lentils. Cover and cook for 10 minutes, stirring often. Stir in the vinegar and capers; cook for 1 minute. Season with salt and pepper. Serve warm or at room temperature, garnished with the cheese.

DINNER

Italian Chicken with Pepper and Onion

SERVES 2

PREP TIME: 10 MINUTES • COOK TIME: 33 MINUTES

TIP: As long as the heat is kept low and you keep stirring, there is no need to use a lot of oil when cooking meat and vegetables.

2 boneless, skinless chicken breast halves (about 4 ounces each)

Salt and black pepper

½ medium onion, thinly sliced

1 red bell pepper, thinly sliced

2 cloves garlic, minced

½ cup reduced-sodium chicken broth

1 tablespoon white wine vinegar

1 teaspoon fresh thyme leaves

4 ounces whole wheat penne or other tube pasta

Preheat the oven to 350°F. Season the chicken with salt and pepper. Lightly coat a medium nonstick skillet with cooking spray; place over medium heat. Brown the chicken for about 4 minutes per side; it will not be cooked through. Transfer to a serving platter.

In the same skillet over medium-low heat, cook the onion and bell pepper for 5 minutes, until softened, stirring. Add the garlic, broth, vinegar, and thyme. Bring to a boil and simmer for 2 minutes, stirring.

Nestle the chicken on top of the vegetables. Transfer the skillet to the oven and bake for 18 minutes, until the chicken is cooked through.

Meanwhile, cook the pasta according to the package directions. Serve with the chicken and vegetables.

Pronto Chicken with Porcini Ragù

SERVES 2

PREP TIME: 10 MINUTES • COOK TIME: 25 MINUTES

Small amounts of sun-dried tomatoes and earthy mushrooms add big flavor to this simple chicken dish. Farro is a hearty, chewy grain that is especially high in fiber and protein. If unavailable, substitute brown rice.

4 ounces farro

½ ounce (about ½ cup) dried porcini mushrooms, rinsed and drained

1 ¼ cups reduced-sodium chicken broth, divided

2 boneless, skinless chicken breast halves (about 4 ounces each), cut in half
     horizontally and pounded to about ¼ inch thick

Salt and black pepper

2 sun-dried tomatoes packed in oil, drained and chopped

½ small shallot, chopped

½ teaspoon red wine vinegar

Cook the farro according to the package directions; keep warm.

Meanwhile, in a medium bowl, combine the mushrooms and 1 cup of the broth (so that the mushrooms are covered). Microwave for 1 minute, then let stand for 5 minutes. Transfer the mushrooms to a cutting board; chop. Return to the bowl with the broth.

Coat a large nonstick skillet with cooking spray; set over medium-high heat. Season the chicken with salt and pepper. Place the chicken in the hot skillet; cook for 2 minutes. Turn over and cook for 1 minute. Transfer to a large plate.

In the same skillet over medium heat, cook the sun-dried tomatoes and shallot for 1 minute, stirring constantly. Add the mushrooms and their broth and the remaining ¼ cup chicken broth. Cook for 4 minutes, stirring to scrape up the browned bits.

Return the chicken and any plate juices to the pan. Cover and simmer for 1 minute, until the chicken is cooked through. Transfer to a clean serving platter. Stir the vinegar into the sauce and season with salt and pepper. Spoon the sauce over the chicken. Serve with the farro.

Seared Striped Bass with Fennel and Orange Salad

SERVES 2

PREP TIME: 5 MINUTES • COOK TIME: 16 MINUTES

Make this dish in the winter months, when oranges are at their best.

TIP: You can substitute red snapper or tilapia for the striped bass.

4 ounces whole wheat spaghetti

2 striped bass fillets (about 5 ounces each)

Salt and black pepper

2 teaspoons olive oil, divided

1 navel orange or large blood orange

1 small fennel bulb, cut in half lengthwise, cored, and very thinly sliced
   crosswise

16 small fresh mint leaves, torn in half

Cook the pasta according to the package directions; keep warm.

Pat the fish dry with paper towels and season with salt and pepper. Add 1 teaspoon of the oil to a medium nonstick skillet; place over medium-high heat. Add the fish to the hot pan, skin side down; cook for 3 minutes, until golden. Turn and cook for 3 minutes, until just cooked through.

Cut the orange into wedges. Working over a medium bowl, remove the segments from the peel, letting the juice fall into the bowl. Toss the segments and juice with the fennel, mint, and remaining 1 teaspoon oil. Season with salt and pepper.

Arrange the fennel and orange salad on 2 serving plates, reserving the dressing in the bowl. Place the bass on top of the salad and spoon some of the dressing over the fish. Serve with the warm spaghetti, drizzling a bit of the dressing over the pasta.

Basque Omelet with Ham and Roasted Pepper

SERVES 2

PREP TIME: 5 MINUTES • COOK TIME: 10 MINUTES

Although called an omelet, this egg dish from the north of Spain is cooked like our scrambled eggs. Serve with toast.

½ cup chopped onion

2 roasted red peppers (from a jar), diced

Salt and black pepper

Pinch of cayenne pepper

4 egg whites, lightly beaten

2 ounces Serrano or deli ham, diced

3 slices whole-grain bread, toasted

Lightly coat a medium nonstick skillet with cooking spray, and place it over medium-low heat. Add the onion: cook for 4 minutes, stirring constantly, until softened. Add roasted peppers, salt and pepper to taste, and cayenne. Cook for 4 minutes, stirring constantly. Transfer to a small bowl.

Wipe out the skillet with a paper towel. Coat the skillet with more cooking spray; place it over low heat until hot.

In a small bowl, whisk the egg whites. Pour them into the hot pan, and cook, stirring constantly, until the eggs are just set. Stir in the pepper mixture and ham. Season with salt and pepper. Serve with the toast.

Spanish Tortilla with Sweet Potatoes

SERVES 2

PREP TIME: 5 MINUTES • COOK TIME: 20 MINUTES

Called a tortilla in Spain, this egg and potato pie is served morning, noon, and night.

½ teaspoon olive oil

1 large sweet potato, unpeeled and diced into small pieces

½ red onion, chopped

2 cloves garlic, chopped

Salt and black pepper

6 egg whites

Salt

2 slices whole-grain bread

Preheat the oven to 350°F. Warm the oil in an ovenproof, medium non-stick skillet over medium-low heat. Add the sweet potato, onion, garlic, and salt and pepper to taste. Cook for 10 minutes, turning the vegetables until they are lightly browned and just tender.

In a medium bowl, whisk the egg whites and salt together. Reduce the heat under the skillet to low; add the eggs to the vegetables and allow them to cook, without stirring, for 5 minutes, until almost set. Transfer the skillet to the oven; bake for 5 minutes until cooked through. Serve with the bread.

LUNCH

Slow-Baked Rice and Beans

SERVES 2

PREP TIME: 5 MINUTES • COOK TIME: 45 MINUTES

Rice and beans are an excellent low-cost source of protein. Here, the rice is baked, as opposed to cooked on the stovetop.

½ cup brown rice

1 can (14 ½ ounces) reduced-sodium chicken broth

Pinch of salt

½ cup drained and rinsed canned black beans, warmed

½ cup halved cherry tomatoes

½ cup fresh cilantro, chopped

Preheat the oven to 375°F. Pour the rice into an 8-inch square glass baking dish or a 2-quart casserole dish.

Combine broth and salt in a glass measuring cup. Bring to a simmer in the microwave. Pour the simmering broth over the rice, stir to combine, then cover the dish tightly with heavy-duty aluminum foil. Bake for 40 to 45 minutes, until the rice is tender and the broth is absorbed. Uncover and fluff the rice with a fork.

Stir the warmed beans and the tomatoes into the rice; garnish with cilantro. Serve.

Pan con Jamón

SERVES 2

PREP TIME: 5 MINUTES

Spaniards are justifiably proud of the ham they produce. If you can find serrano ham, use it to make this open-faced sandwich. If unavailable, you can use any ham, or smoked turkey for a change of pace.

2 tomatoes, halved

Salt

½ small (about 8 inches) whole-grain baguette, halved lengthwise

1 teaspoon extra-virgin olive oil

4 thin slices serrano or other ham (about 3 ounces each)

Baby lettuce or romaine lettuce, torn

Place a grater over a bowl. Rub the cut sides of the tomato halves over the grater until the flesh is grated. Discard the skins. Season the tomato pulp with salt.

Using your fingers, scoop out some of the soft insides of the baguette, creating a channel in each half. Toast the remaining bread. Spoon the tomato pulp into the channels of the toast. Drizzle with olive oil and top with a slice of ham and some lettuce. Serve.

SNACK

Red Lentil Purée

SERVES 4 (2 CUPS)

PREP TIME: 5 MINUTES • COOK TIME: 12 MINUTES

This hearty dip makes enough for 4 servings. It will keep, for up to a
week refrigerated. Serve warm or at room temperature with pita bread
and veggies for dipping.

  1 cup red lentils washed and picked over

  1 cup reduced-sodium chicken broth

  Salt and black pepper

  3 tablespoons fresh lemon juice

  1 teaspoon chopped fresh thyme

  Celery stalks, for dipping

In a small saucepan over medium-high heat, combine lentils, broth, and
salt and pepper to taste; bring to a boil. Reduce heat to low; cover and
simmer for 12 minutes, until softened.

In a food processor, combine lentils, lemon juice, and thyme. Process
until smooth. Serve with celery stalks.

Winter Salad with Clementines and Homemade Sherry-Wine Vinaigrette

SERVES 2

PREP TIME: 5 MINUTES

Spaniards usually toss red onion in their salads. If raw onion bothers your stomach, feel free to leave it out.

2 teaspoons sherry wine or red wine vinegar

1 teaspoon extra-virgin olive oil

2 clementines, peeled and divided into wedges

Salt and black pepper

2 cups baby arugula

1 small head radicchio, halved and torn into pieces (about 5 cups loosely
     packed)

2 tablespoons thinly sliced red onion

1 cup shredded cooked chicken breast meat

In a small bowl, combine and whisk the vinegar and olive oil. Squeeze the juice of 1 clementine segment into the bowl so that it adds to the dressing. Season with salt and pepper.

In a large serving bowl, combine the arugula, radicchio, and onion. Add the remaining clementine segments and shredded chicken. Add the vinaigrette and toss to coat. Serve.

Tuna-Stuffed Tomatoes

SERVES 2

PREP TIME: 5 MINUTES

Toast a couple of slices of whole-grain bread, then cut them into triangles to serve with these tuna-stuffed tomatoes.

6 ounces canned solid albacore tuna, packed in water and drained

1 tablespoon finely chopped red onion

½ small cucumber, peeled and chopped

2 tablespoons fat-free mayonnaise

2 tablespoons fresh lemon juice

Salt

2 medium tomatoes

4 tablespoons chopped fresh tarragon

2 slices whole-grain bread, toasted

In a medium bowl, toss the tuna, onion, and cucumber. Add mayonnaise, lemon juice, and salt to taste.

Using a paring knife, cut a big hole in the tomatoes, creating a cavity for the tuna salad. Spoon the tuna mixture into the tomatoes, allowing the tuna to mound on top. Sprinkle with the tarragon. Serve immediately with toasted bread.

Citrus Tuna Ceviche with Lime Chips

SERVES 2

PREP TIME: 10 MINUTES (PLUS MARINADING) • COOK TIME: 15 MINUTES

With ceviche, the fish actually "cooks" in the citrus marinade. The fish may be marinated a day in advance, but after about 4 hours, drain the juice from the fish. Wait to add the tomato and cilantro until just before serving.

TIP: You can bake the chips up to 2 days in advance.

⅓ pound fresh yellowfin tuna, diced into ½-inch pieces

¼ cup fresh lime juice

¼ cup fresh lemon juice

2 scallions, finely chopped

1 jalapeño, seeded and finely chopped

1 tomato, diced into ½-inch pieces

¼ cup chopped fresh cilantro

Salt

Lime tortilla chips (see below)

In a nonreactive bowl, combine the tuna, lime juice, lemon juice, and scallions. There should be enough juice to fully cover the fish. Cover and refrigerate for about 4 hours until a cube of fish no longer looks raw when cut into. Drain out the juices.

Add jalapeno, tomato, and cilantro, and season with salt. Cover and refrigerate if not serving immediately. Serve with the chips.

Lime Tortilla Chips: Preheat the oven to 350°F. Cut I whole-grain tortilla into 8 wedges. In a small cup, combine 2 teaspoons of fresh lime juice with ¼ teaspoon of olive oil. Arrange the wedges on a baking sheet, and brush their tops with the lime-oil combination. Sprinkle with salt. Bake for 12 minutes until crisp.

Garbanzo Bean Stew with Escarole

SERVES 2

PREP TIME: 5 MINUTES • COOK TIME: 30 MINUTES

Meaty garbanzo beans add protein and fiber to this classic Mediterranean stew.

½ teaspoon olive oil

½ small onion, chopped

2 cloves garlic, finely chopped

Salt and black pepper

7 ounces (½ can) garbanzo beans (chickpeas), drained

1 cup reduced-sodium chicken broth

2 teaspoons chopped fresh thyme or 1 teaspoon dried

¼ teaspoon crumbled saffron

1 cup thinly sliced escarole (about ½ head)

Warm the oil in a pot over medium heat. Add the onion, garlic, and salt and pepper to taste; cook 5 minutes, stirring constantly. Add the beans, broth, ¼ cup water, thyme, and saffron, and bring all to a boil. Reduce the heat and cook for 20 minutes.

Remove half of the stew; purée it in a blender or food processor. Return the purée to the pot. (Alternatively, you may use an immersion blender briefly to purée the stew directly in the pot.) Add the escarole. Simmer for 5 minutes until the escarole is tender, adding more water if the mixture is too thick.

Ladle the stew into bowls to serve, and season with salt and pepper to taste.

DINNER

Seared Striped Sea Bass on a Bed of Lentils

SERVES 2

PREP TIME: 10 MINUTES • COOK TIME: 38 MINUTES

This restaurant-style dinner is deceptively simple to make.

TIP: Sherry wine vinegar is a typical Spanish vinegar. If unavailable, substitute red wine vinegar.

Lentils

2 carrots, cut into small dice

1 stalk celery, cut into small dice

½ small yellow onion, chopped

2 teaspoons chopped fresh thyme, or ½ teaspoon dried

1 cup green or brown lentils, washed and picked over

2 cups reduced-sodium chicken broth

2 teaspoon sherry wine vinegar

Salt and black pepper

See Bass

2 striped sea bass fillets (4 ounce each), with skin

½ teaspoon olive oil

2 tablespoons chopped fresh flat-leaf parsley

1½ cups cooked brown rice, warmed

To cook the lentils, lightly coat a medium nonstick skillet or Dutch oven with cooking spray and place it over medium heat. Add the carrots, celery, onion, and thyme; cook for 6 minutes, stirring constantly, until softened. Stir in the lentils and broth; bring it to a boil. Cover and reduce the heat to low to simmer for 30 minutes the until the lentils are tender. Stir in the vinegar. Season with salt and pepper.

To cook the fish, pat the fillets dry with a paper towel; season them with salt and pepper. Warm the oil in a medium ovenproof skillet over medium-high heat until it is hot but not smoking. Add the fillets, skin side down. Cook for 4 minutes, until golden brown. Turn the fillets and cook for 4 more minutes until just cooked through. Ladle the lentils into shallow serving bowls. Place fish on top of the lentils and garnish with the parsley. Serve with the rice.

Family-Style Pollo en Salse de Tomate

SERVES 2

PREP TIME: 10 MINUTES • COOK TIME: 22 MINUTES

Many Spanish dishes start with a "sofrito," made with tomatoes, onions, mushrooms, and green pepper. Here, the sauce combines with pan-seared chicken for a quick and easy main course.

½ medium yellow onion, chopped

3 cloves garlic, chopped

½ green bell pepper, chopped

3 white mushrooms, thickly sliced

1 can (15 ounces) diced tomatoes

2 boneless, skinless chicken breast halves (about 4 ounces each)

Salt and black pepper

1½ cups cooked brown rice, warmed

Lightly coat a large nonstick skillet with cooking spray and place it over medium heat. Add the onion, garlic, bell pepper, mushrooms, and a splash of the tomato sauce from the canned tomatoes. Cook for 5 minutes, stirring often. Add the tomatoes. Cook for 6 minutes, stirring often. If the sauce seems too thick, add a bit of water. Retain some sauce in the pan.

Lightly coat a medium nonstick skillet with cooking spray. Season the chicken with salt and pepper, and add it to the hot pan. Cook for 5 minutes per side. The chicken will not be cooked through. Cut the chicken into ½-inch-thick diagonal slices.

Arrange the chicken slices in the warm sauce in the skillet over low heat. Gently coat the chicken with the sauce; cover the pan and cook over low heat for 6 minutes. Season with salt and pepper and serve over the rice.

Saffron Shrimp Paella

SERVES 2

PREP TIME: 10 MINUTES • COOK TIME: 23 MINUTES

Paella is arguably the most famous dish of Spain. It can be made with fish, chicken, or sausage, and sometimes is made with all three.

½ teaspoon olive oil

1 small onion, chopped

½ red bell pepper, chopped

3 cloves garlic, chopped

¼ teaspoon saffron threads, crumbled

¼ teaspoon hot Spanish paprika or hot Hungarian paprika

Salt and black pepper

1 can (14 ½ ounces) reduced-sodium chicken broth, plus more if needed

¾ cup arborio rice

6 ounces peeled, deveined large shrimp (uncooked or thawed cooked frozen)

½ cup frozen small peas, thawed

In a medium heavy skillet with 2-inch sides, warm the oil over medium heat. Add the onion and bell pepper. Cook for 6 minutes until softened, stirring often. Stir in the garlic, saffron, paprika, and salt and pepper to taste. Add broth and rice.

Bring to a boil; reduce the heat to low; cover and simmer for 12 minutes until the rice is almost tender. Nestle the shrimp and peas in the rice, and add ¼ cup (or more) of the broth to moisten. Cover and cook until the shrimp are just opaque in the center, about 5 minutes. Season to taste with salt and pepper. Serve.

BREAKFAST

Gaeran Mari

SERVES 1

PREP TIME: 5 MINUTES • COOK TIME: 2 MINUTES

This Korean rolled egg dish is as easy to make as an American omelet. We fill out the meal and increase the fiber by serving it with a side of warm brown rice.

TIP: Look for instant brown rice at your market.

4 egg whites

¼ cup finely chopped onions

¼ cup finely chopped carrots

Salt and black pepper

1 sheet Korean roasted seaweed or nori

¾ cup cooked brown rice, warmed

Coat a medium nonstick skillet with cooking spray; place over medium-low heat. In a medium bowl, whisk the egg whites, onion, carrot, and salt and pepper to taste until well combined. Pour into the warm skillet; cook for 1 minute, until almost cooked through. Place the seaweed on top of the eggs; cook for 1 minute until just set. Run a rubber spatula around the edges of the omelet to loosen from the pan. Lift one edge and carefully slide the omelet onto a cutting board. Roll up tight and cut into 1-inch slices. Transfer to a serving plate and serve with the rice.

Chicken Noodle Soup

SERVES 2

PREP TIME: 5 MINUTES • COOK TIME: 8 MINUTES

Hot noodle soup is often served for breakfast in Korea. Save time by using preshredded carrots and the meat from a rotisserie chicken.

TIP: Cellophane noodles, also called glass or mung bean noodles, are typical Korean noodles. If unavailable, substitute soba or udon noodles.

3 ounces cellophane or soba noodles

3 cups reduced-sodium chicken broth

1 tablespoon reduced-sodium soy sauce

½ teaspoon Chinese five-spice powder

¾ cup shredded carrots

1 ½ cups shredded cooked chicken breast

3 scallions, thinly sliced

Cook the noodles according to the package directions; drain.

Place a medium saucepan over high heat. Add the broth, soy sauce, and five-spice powder; stir to combine. Add the carrots; cook for 3 minutes. Add the cooked noodles and chicken; cook until warmed through. Serve in deep bowls, garnished with the scallions.

Sesame Rice Bowl

SERVES 1

PREP TIME: 5 MINUTES • COOK TIME: 40 MINUTES

A hot rice bowl, either laden with veggies and spices or simply flavored with soy and spinach, is a popular breakfast or snack in Korea.

2 egg whites, lightly beaten

⅓ cup brown rice

1 tablespoon minced scallion (white part only)

Salt and black pepper

1 cup reduced-sodium chicken or beef broth

3 cups baby spinach

1 teaspoon Asian sesame oil

2 teaspoons reduced-sodium soy sauce

Lightly coat a small nonstick saucepan with cooking spray; place over medium heat. Add the egg whites; cook until scrambled, stirring. Transfer to a plate.

Wipe out the skillet with a paper towel. Coat again with cooking spray and place over medium heat. Add the rice, scallion, and salt and pepper to taste; stir for 30 seconds to coat the rice. Add the broth and ¼ cup water; bring to a simmer. Reduce the heat to low, cover, and cook for 40 minutes, until cooked through. In the last 2 minutes of cooking, stir in the spinach until wilted. Stir in the scrambled egg whites.

Transfer the rice and spinach to a serving bowl. Toss with the sesame oil and soy sauce; serve.

LUNCH

BBQ Beef Rice Bowl

SERVES 2

PREP TIME: 5 MINUTES • COOK TIME: 8 MINUTES

Koreans are known for their barbecue, especially barbecued beef, and Korean barbecue sauce is now available in the United States. It's a combination of sake, soy sauce, and garlic. If you can't find it, use a combination of these three ingredients to equal 3 tablespoons.

6 ounces flank steak, very thinly sliced

3 tablespoons Korean barbecue sauce

4 ounces green beans, trimmed and chopped on the diagonal

½ cup shredded carrots

Salt

1 ½ cups cooked brown rice, warmed

1 scallion, thinly sliced

In a medium bowl, combine the steak and barbecue sauce.

Coat a medium nonstick skillet with cooking spray; set over medium-high heat. Add the beans and carrots and salt to taste; stir-fry for 2 minutes. Add ¼ cup water; cover and cook for 3 minutes, just until tender. Remove to a plate.

Increase the heat under the skillet to high. Add the beef and sauce; stir-fry for 2 minutes, until the meat is no longer pink. Add the vegetables; cook for 1 minute to warm through.

Scoop the rice into 2 serving bowls and add the beef mixture. Garnish with the scallion and serve.

Southeast Asian Shrimp Salad

SERVES 2

PREP TIME: 10 MINUTES

Use frozen shrimp for this recipe. Just double-check that the package indicates that the shrimp are cooked.

Dressing

2 tablespoons sesame-ginger dressing

½ teaspoon Asian hot chili paste sauce, such as sambal oelek

Salad

4 ounces frozen cooked (peeled and deveined) medium shrimp, thawed

½ cucumber, peeled and cubed

1 cup thinly sliced Chinese (napa) cabbage

½ red bell pepper, thinly sliced

2 scallions, thinly sliced

1 tablespoon chopped peanuts

1 ½ cups cooked brown rice, warmed

To make the dressing, in a small bowl whisk the sesame-ginger dressing and the chili paste until blended.

To make the salad, in a medium bowl combine the shrimp, cucumber, cabbage, bell pepper, and scallions. Toss with the dressing and sprinkle with the peanuts. Serve with the rice.

Crisp Vegetable Salad

SERVES 2

PREP TIME: 5 MINUTES • COOK TIME: 5 MINUTES

This is a filling snack for a hot day. Use this recipe as a starting point—add or substitute your favorite veggies or those that are in season.

1 large carrot

½ red bell pepper, quartered lengthwise

8 sugar snap peas

½ cup frozen shelled edamame, thawed

1 ½ teaspoons sesame oil

2 teaspoons white wine vinegar

1 teaspoon fresh lemon juice

Salt and black pepper

Pinch of red pepper flakes or powdered red chiles (*kochukaru*), optional

Handful of pea shoots or alfalfa sprouts

Using a vegetable peeler, peel long strips from the carrot. Slice the bell pepper and sugar snap peas lengthwise into very thin strips.

Cook the edamame according to the package directions.

In a medium serving bowl, whisk the oil, vinegar, lemon juice, salt and pepper to taste, and the pepper flakes. Add the sliced vegetables, edamame, and pea shoots. Toss until thoroughly coated and serve.

Ginger Chicken Lettuce Wrap

SERVES 2

PREP TIME: 5 MINUTES • COOK TIME: 6 MINUTES

Be sure to use light coconut milk, not the super-thick coconut cream. Also be sure to use Asian sesame oil—a dark, thick, intensely flavored oil—not the light sesame oil generally used for cooking.

3 tablespoons unsweetened light coconut milk

1 teaspoon peeled and minced fresh ginger

1 tablespoon reduced-sodium soy sauce

½ teaspoon Asian sesame oil

4 ounces thinly sliced boneless, skinless chicken breast halves (cutlets),
    sliced crosswise into ¼-inch-wide strips

4 lettuce leaves

⅓ cup canned lentils, drained and rinsed

Lime wedges

In a food processor, combine the coconut milk, ginger, soy sauce, and sesame oil; process until smooth. Pour into a plastic bowl and add the chicken strips. Marinate in the refrigerator for at least 15 minutes.

Thread the chicken strips onto 10-inch skewers, straightening the pieces as much as possible. Lightly coat a grill pan or nonstick skillet with cooking spray; place over medium-high heat.

Add the chicken; cook for 3 minutes per side, until cooked through.

Place the lettuce leaves on the countertop; remove the chicken from the skewers. Fill each lettuce leaf with some chicken and lentils. Squeeze fresh lime juice over the lentils, fold over the lettuce, and serve.

Seaweed Salad with Edamame

SERVES 2

PREP TIME: 5 MINUTES • COOK TIME: 5 MINUTES

Look for wakame seaweed in the freezer or refrigerated section of a Japanese or specialty market. This packaged fresh seaweed is sold salted, so it's important to rinse it several times before using.

2/3 cup frozen shelled edamame, thawed

1 cup (2 ounces) wakame

1 tablespoon rice vinegar

1 teaspoon fresh lemon juice

1 teaspoon peeled and minced fresh ginger

1 teaspoon reduced-sodium soy sauce

Cook the edamame according to the package directions.

Soak the seaweed in warm water for 5 minutes. Rinse in three or four changes of cold water, swishing it around to release the salt. Drain, then squeeze between clean kitchen towels to remove any excess moisture.

In a medium bowl, whisk the vinegar, lemon juice, ginger, and soy sauce. Add the seaweed and edamame; toss to coat. Serve.

Shrimp and Black Bean Fried Rice

SERVES 2

PREP TIME: 5 MINUTES • COOK TIME: 7 MINUTES

Use frozen shrimp for convenience. Precooked brown rice, sold frozen at health food stores, is another great product for quick cooking.

½ small onion, chopped

1 egg white, lightly beaten

1 teaspoon peeled and minced fresh ginger

1 small green chile, seeded and chopped

4 ounces frozen precooked (peeled and deveined) small shrimp, thawed

¾ cup cooked brown rice

¼ cup canned black beans, drained and rinsed

2 tablespoons fresh lemon juice

Lightly coat a wok or deep nonstick skillet with cooking spray; place over medium heat. Add the onion; cook for 3 minutes, until softened. Add the egg white; cook for 1 minute without stirring. Using a wooden spoon, fold the egg white over so that it cooks through. Scrape the egg-onion mixture onto a platter.

Coat the pan again with cooking spray; set over medium heat. Stir in the ginger and chile; cook for 30 seconds, stirring. Add the shrimp; cook for 2 minutes. Stir in the rice, beans, and egg mixture; cook to warm through. Divide between 2 serving plates. Drizzle with the lemon juice and serve.

DINNER

Chicken and Sweet Potato Stir-Fry

SERVES 2

PREP TIME: 10 MINUTES • COOK TIME: 13 MINUTES

One serving of this satisfying supper provides more than 400 percent of your daily vitamin A needs.

1 small sweet potato (about 8 ounces), unpeeled, cut crosswise into
    ⅓-inch-thick rounds, then cut into thin strips

½ small red onion, very thinly sliced

8 ounces thinly sliced boneless, skinless chicken breast halves (cutlets),
    sliced crosswise into ¼-inch-wide strips

Salt and black pepper

1 tablespoon peeled and minced fresh ginger

2 cloves garlic, minced

1 cup shredded cabbage or coleslaw mix

1 tablespoon plus 1 teaspoon hoisin sauce

Lightly coat a large nonstick skillet with cooking spray; place over medium-high heat. Add the sweet potato and onion; cook for 8 minutes, until softened, stirring and adding water if the mixture seems dry.

Season the chicken with salt and pepper. Coat the skillet again with cooking spray; place over medium heat. Add the chicken, ginger, and garlic; stir-fry for 2 minutes. Add the cabbage; stir-fry for 3 minutes, until the chicken is cooked through and the cabbage is wilted but still crunchy. Stir in the hoisin sauce and 2 tablespoons water until warmed through. Serve.

Korean Beef Grill

SERVES 2

PREP TIME: 5 MINUTES • COOK TIME: 3 MINUTES

Here's a typical recipe for *bibimbap,* or Korean barbecue. The savory grilled beef is served wrapped up in lettuce leaves with rice.

TIP: Clean the lettuce leaves thoroughly and keep as whole leaves. They will serve as a cup to hold the spicy beef mixture.

7 ounces flank steak, very thinly sliced

2 tablespoons Korean barbecue sauce (or 2 tablespoons reduced-sodium
    soy sauce, 2 minced garlic cloves, and 1 tablespoon rice vinegar)

½ very ripe pear, peeled, cored, and minced

2 teaspoons peeled and minced fresh ginger

Salt and black pepper

1 red bell pepper, thinly sliced

1½ cups cooked brown rice, warmed

6 romaine lettuce leaves, rinsed and patted dry

Reduced-sodium soy sauce

In a large resealable plastic bag, combine the steak, barbecue sauce, pear, ginger, and salt and pepper to taste; turn to coat. Refrigerate for 2 hours.

Remove the beef from the marinade, discard the marinade.

Preheat the grill or a nonstick grill pan lightly coated with cooking spray over high heat. Add the beef; grill for 3 minutes, or until done, stirring often.

Drop one-quarter of the meat mixture, a few pepper slices, and some rice into a lettuce cup. Drizzle with soy sauce and fold into a package. (Alternatively, you can dip the whole lettuce package into soy sauce.) Repeat with the remaining leaves and serve.

Classic Home-Style Korean Stir-Fry

SERVES 2

PREP TIME: 10 MINUTES • COOK TIME: 10 MINUTES

Although Koreans often cook with cellophane noodles, you can substitute whatever Asian noodles you can find. Use the meat from a rotisserie chicken for a quick dinner.

4 ounces cellophane or udon noodles

1 small onion, thinly sliced

3 cloves garlic, finely chopped

4 ounces baby spinach

3 scallions, chopped

3 shiitake mushrooms, stemmed, wiped clean, and sliced

1 cooked boneless, skinless chicken breast half (about 4 ounces), shredded

2 tablespoons reduced-sodium soy sauce

1 teaspoon Asian sesame oil

Cook the noodles according to the package directions. Drain and rinse under cold water to prevent sticking.

Coat a large nonstick skillet with cooking spray; place over medium-high heat. Add the onion and garlic; cook for 1 minute, stirring. Add the spinach, scallions, and mushrooms; cook for 4 minutes, stirring. The vegetables should still be crispy.

Reduce the heat to low. Add the cooked noodles, chicken, soy sauce, and sesame oil. Cook for 2 minutes, tossing to combine the flavors and warm through. Serve.

Yogurt with Apricot and Pomegranate

SERVES 1

PREP TIME: 5 MINUTES

Apricots and pomegranates are popular fruits in Israel. In the winter months, look for cartons of pomegranate seeds in the produce section of your supermarket.

- 1 cup nonfat plain Greek yogurt
- 1 tablespoon agave nectar
- 1 apricot, peeled and pitted, and cut into wedges
- 4 tablespoons pomegranate seeds
- ¼ cup chopped natural almonds

Spoon the yogurt into a medium bowl; stir in the agave nectar. Top with the apricot wedges, pomegranate seeds, and almonds. Serve.

Warm Pita with Yogurt and Dill

SERVES 1

PREP TIME: 5 MINUTES

Now that cherry tomatoes are available year-round, you can enjoy this savory breakfast anytime. More good news: this little dish contains more than the daily requirement of vitamins A and C.

3/4 cup nonfat plain Greek yogurt

2 tablespoons chopped fresh dill

1 teaspoon fresh lemon juice

6 cherry tomatoes, quartered

1 whole-grain pita

In a medium bowl, combine the yogurt, dill, lemon juice, and tomatoes.

Warm the pita in the oven or toaster oven; cut into wedges. Use the wedges to scoop up the yogurt mixture.

Warm Cinnamon Bulgur with Nuts and Berries

SERVES 1

PREP TIME: 5 MINUTES • COOK TIME: 15 MINUTES

Tired of oatmeal? Try hearty, rich-in-fiber bulgur instead. This grain is very popular in the Middle East.

1 ¼ cups nonfat milk

½ cup light bulgur (cracked wheat)

1 teaspoon agave nectar

½ teaspoon ground cinnamon

½ cup fresh raspberries

1 tablespoon toasted chopped walnuts

Place a small saucepan over heat. Add the milk and bring to just a simmer. Reduce the heat to low. Stir in the bulgur; simmer for 12 minutes, until most of the liquid is absorbed and the grain is just tender, stirring often. Remove from the heat; cover and let rest for 5 minutes.

Spoon the bulgur into a serving bowl. Stir in the agave nectar, cinnamon, and berries. Top with the nuts and serve.

LUNCH

Fresh Herb Falafel

SERVES 4

PREP TIME: 5 MINUTES • COOK TIME: 10 MINUTES

Falafel is a very popular street food sold throughout the Middle East. Here it's served atop chopped romaine lettuce with a dollop of tzatziki.

TIP: Wrap and refrigerate any leftover falafel for a quick lunch to bring to work.

1 can (12 to 14 ounces) chickpeas, drained and rinsed

¼ cup minced red onion

¼ cup whole wheat bread crumbs

⅓ cup fresh flat-leaf parsley leaves

⅓ cup fresh cilantro leaves

1 teaspoon ground cumin

2 teaspoons canola oil

Romaine lettuce leaves

1 cup tzatziki (see recipe page 249)

In a food processor, combine the chickpeas, onion, bread crumbs, parsley, cilantro, and cumin. Process until it has the consistency of a thick paste. Shape into rounded patties about the size of a Ping-Pong ball; slightly flatten.

Place the oil in a medium nonstick skillet over medium heat. When the oil is hot, cook the falafel for about 10 minutes, until golden and semi-firm, turning often to ensure even browning.

Arrange the lettuce leaves on 4 serving plates. Top with the falafel and tzatziki; serve.

Roasted Tomato Quinoa with Fresh Herbs and Thick Yogurt

SERVES 2

PREP TIME: 10 MINUTES • COOK TIME: 55 MINUTES

Make this meal on a Sunday evening, since you'll need some cooking time. (Fortunately, nearly all the time is unattended.) Although this dish is traditionally made with couscous, we've substituted quinoa for the added fiber and protein.

TIP: Greek yogurt, because of its thick consistency, is essential to this recipe.

6 ounces grape or cherry tomatoes, cut in half lengthwise

3 cloves garlic, unpeeled

1 teaspoon olive oil

1 tablespoon fresh lemon juice

Salt and black pepper

$^2/_3$ cup quinoa

Reduced-sodium chicken broth (check quinoa package directions for amount)

$^1/_2$ cup chopped fresh flat-leaf parsley

2 tablespoons chopped fresh mint

$^1/_4$ cup nonfat plain Greek yogurt

Preheat the oven to 250°F. Arrange the tomatoes cut side up in one layer in a large baking pan. Add the garlic. Roast for 45 minutes, until the tomatoes are slightly shriveled around the edges.

Squeeze the roasted garlic into the bowl of a food processor or blender. Add the oil, 1 tablespoon water, the lemon juice, salt and pepper to taste, and ½ cup of the roasted tomatoes. Purée until the dressing is very smooth.

Cook the quinoa according to the package directions, substituting chicken broth for the water. Transfer to a bowl and stir in the roasted tomato dressing, remaining roasted tomatoes, parsley, mint, and salt and pepper to taste. Serve topped with the yogurt.

Spicy Lamb and Feta Pita Pizzas

SERVES 2

PREP TIME: 10 MINUTES • COOK TIME: 15 MINUTES

Since feta is a strongly flavored cheese, you don't need to add a lot for these colorful pizzas to pack a powerful punch.

4 ounces extra-lean ground lamb

½ teaspoon ground allspice

½ teaspoon dried oregano, crumbled

Salt and black pepper

2 whole-grain pitas

1 red bell pepper, chopped

2 ounces fat-free feta cheese, crumbled

2 tablespoons chopped fresh mint

Preheat the oven to 400°F. Warm a baking sheet in the oven.

Coat a medium nonstick skillet with cooking spray; place over medium heat. Add the lamb; cook for 5 minutes, until cooked through and browned, breaking up the meat as it cooks. Drain all the fat from the skillet. Stir in the allspice, oregano, and salt and pepper to taste.

Place the pitas on the countertop. Sprinkle evenly with the lamb mixture, bell pepper, and cheese. Using a spatula, transfer to the hot baking sheet. Bake for 10 minutes, until the cheese melts and the crust is crisp. Garnish with the mint and serve.

SNACK

Lemon and Parsley Hummus

MAKES 2 CUPS

PREP TIME: 5 MINUTES

Serve this creamy dip with carrot and celery sticks. Believe it or not, ¼ cup contains almost half your daily iron requirement.

TIP: This is a great recipe for a small party, as it makes enough for 8 servings. It also will keep in the refrigerator for a week, so it makes for a super-healthy snack.

1 can (12–14 ounces) chickpeas, rinsed and drained, divided

1 clove garlic, minced

¼ cup fresh lemon juice

¼ cup well-stirred tahini

½ teaspoon ground cumin

Salt

1 ½ cups fresh flat-leaf parsley leaves

In a food processor, purée ½ cup of the chickpeas and the garlic until the garlic is minced. Add ½ cup water, the lemon juice, tahini, cumin, salt to taste, and remaining chickpeas; purée until smooth. Add the parsley; purée until smooth. Transfer to a bowl, cover, and refrigerate until serving. Store in a covered container in the refrigerator for up to 1 week.

Warm Lavash with Sun-Dried Tomatoes and Creamy Herb Spread

SERVES 2

PREP TIME: 5 MINUTES • COOK TIME: 5 MINUTES

Lavash is a common Middle Eastern flatbread. If it's unavailable, substitute whole wheat pita bread. The creamy spread features fresh green herbs—an essential component of Israeli cuisine.

½ cup chopped fresh flat-leaf parsley

¼ cup chopped fresh basil

2 tablespoons chopped fresh chives

2 tablespoons fresh lemon juice

1 ½ ounces reduced-fat cream cheese, at room temperature

⅓ cup nonfat plain Greek yogurt

Salt and black pepper

1 whole-grain lavash or pita

1 cup sun-dried tomatoes packed in oil, drained and chopped

1 cup chopped romaine lettuce

In a blender or food processor, process the parsley, basil, chives, lemon juice, and cream cheese until blended. Add the yogurt; blend until combined. Season with salt and pepper to taste. Cover and refrigerate until serving.

Warm the lavash in the oven or microwave. Assemble the wrap: slather the bread with the herb spread, add the chopped tomatoes and lettuce, and fold the bread over. Cut in half and serve.

Roasted Garlic Baba Ghanoush

MAKES 2 CUPS

PREP TIME: 10 MINUTES • COOK TIME: 35 MINUTES

Baba ghanoush is a popular dish throughout the Middle East. It's usually used as a dip, but it's also delicious in sandwiches or as a garnish. Note that this recipe makes enough to serve 6.

1 medium eggplant

2 cloves garlic, unpeeled

¼ cup well-stirred tahini

¼ cup fresh lemon juice

½ cup canned white kidney or cannellini beans, drained and rinsed

Salt

½ whole-grain pita for each serving

Preheat the oven to 400°F. Using a fork, pierce the eggplant in several places. Wrap the garlic in foil. Place the eggplant and garlic on a baking sheet; roast for 35 minutes, turning a few times, until the eggplant is soft. Remove from the oven and let cool.

Cut the eggplant in half lengthwise. Scrape the flesh into the bowl of a food processor. Squeeze the roasted garlic into the bowl. Add the tahini, lemon juice, beans, and salt to taste. Purée until smooth. Cover and refrigerate before serving with the pita.

Sautéed Shallot Spinach with Brown Rice

SERVES 2

PREP TIME: 5 MINUTES • COOK TIME: 5 MINUTES

Using cooked rice and a bag of spinach makes for a quick snack. Look for cooked brown rice in the freezer section of your market.

TIP: Spinach really cooks down as it wilts. Add the leaves to the pot gradually.

½ teaspoon olive oil

½ shallot, minced

2 cloves garlic, chopped

1 bag (8 to 10 ounces) spinach

¾ cup cooked brown rice or brown and wild rice mix

Salt and black pepper

3 ounces fat-free feta cheese, crumbled

Warm the oil in a medium nonstick saucepan over medium-low heat. Add the shallot and garlic; cook for 1 minute, stirring. Add the spinach and ¾ cup water; cover and cook for 4 minutes, until the water evaporates and the spinach is wilted, stirring. Stir in the rice to warm through; season with salt and pepper. Spoon into 2 serving bowls, garnish with the feta, and serve.

DINNER

Grilled Lemon Chicken with Spiced Couscous

SERVES 2

PREP TIME: 5 MINUTES (PLUS MARINADING) • COOK TIME: 24 MINUTES

Although there are many spices in this dish, the meal comes together quickly. Here we use the traditional, high-fiber bulgur to make the couscous side dish.

Couscous

½ cup bulgur

Reduced-sodium chicken broth (check bulgur package directions for
    amount)

1 tablespoon peeled and minced fresh ginger

¼ teaspoon ground turmeric

¼ teaspoon ground cinnamon

¼ teaspoon ground cumin

½ red bell pepper, cut into small dice

2 tablespoons fresh lemon juice

Salt and black pepper

Chicken

2 tablespoons fresh lemon juice

Salt and black pepper

2 boneless, skinless chicken breast halves (about 4 ounces each)

To make the couscous, prepare the bulgur according to the package directions, substituting broth for the water and adding the ginger, turmeric, cinnamon, and cumin.

In a medium bowl, combine the cooked bulgur, bell pepper, lemon juice, and salt and pepper to taste.

To make the chicken, place the lemon juice and salt and pepper to taste in a large resealable plastic bag. Add the chicken, seal the bag, and turn to coat. Let marinate for 10 minutes.

Preheat the grill or a nonstick grill pan, lightly coated with cooking spray over medium-high heat. Add the chicken; grill for 6 minutes per side, until just cooked through. Mound the couscous on 2 serving plates and top with the chicken. Serve.

Lamb and Tomato Stew

SERVES 2

PREP TIME: 15 MINUTES • COOK TIME: 1¼ HOURS

Serve this hearty, rich stew on a cold winter night.

TIP: When searing meat, it's imperative to use a heavy pot, or the meat will burn. Watch the flame under the meat; if the lamb seems to be burning, lower the heat. You want it to be lightly browned, not cooked through.

> 2 teaspoons canola or olive oil
>
> 7 ounces lamb stew meat, cut into 1-inch pieces
>
> Salt and black pepper
>
> ³/₄ cup red wine, divided
>
> 1 small onion, sliced
>
> 3 cloves garlic, minced
>
> 1 teaspoon dried rosemary
>
> 1 can (15 ounces) Italian-style tomatoes, drained and crushed
>
> ³/₄ cup frozen petit peas, thawed

Warm the oil in a heavy medium saucepan or Dutch oven over medium-high heat. Season the lamb with salt and pepper. Add half the lamb to the pan; cook for about 2 minutes, turning the pieces until browned. The meat will not be cooked through. Transfer to a platter.

Add ¼ cup of the wine to the pot, stirring for 1 minute to scrape up the browned bits. Empty the bits and any liquid in the pot onto the plate with the meat. Repeat the process with the remaining lamb and another ¼ cup wine.

To the same pot over medium-low heat, add the onion, garlic, rosemary, and remaining ¼ cup wine; cook for 4 minutes, stirring. Add the tomatoes, lamb, and any plate juices. Increase the heat and bring to a boil. Cover, reduce the heat to medium-low, and simmer for about 1 hour, until the lamb is tender. Add up to 1 cup water during the cooking time to prevent the stew from getting too dry. Add the peas; cook for 5 minutes, until cooked through. Serve.

Spinach Omelet with Two Cheeses

SERVES 2

PREP TIME: 5 MINUTES • COOK TIME: 9 MINUTES

Using a bag of prewashed baby spinach means there's no trimming or chopping. Just remember to add the leaves gradually to the skillet—they will cook down quickly.

4 ounces baby spinach

2 tablespoons part-skim ricotta cheese

6 egg whites

Salt and black pepper

2 tablespoons crumbled reduced-fat feta cheese

Lightly coat a medium nonstick skillet with cooking spray; place over medium-low heat. Gradually add the spinach and ¼ cup water; cook for 4 minutes, until the water evaporates and the spinach is wilted, stirring occasionally. Transfer to a medium bowl and stir in the ricotta.

In another medium bowl, whisk the egg whites and salt and pepper to taste.

Wipe out the skillet with a paper towel and coat again with cooking spray. Place over medium heat until hot. Add the egg whites; cook for 3 *seconds,* until the edges start to set. Using a spatula, draw the cooked egg to the center of the pan. Tilt the pan so the uncooked egg runs underneath the cooked part. Repeat all around the edge of the pan until the omelet is just set.

Drop the spinach mixture onto one half of the omelet and sprinkle with the feta. Cook for 10 *seconds,* until the desired doneness. Run the spatula around the omelet to loosen the edge. Jerk the pan sharply to move the entire omelet. Tilt the pan, resting the edge on a serving plate. Gently roll the omelet onto the plate, using the spatula to fold it over the filling. Serve.

Fresh Fruit Salad with Yogurt

SERVES 2

PREP TIME: 5 MINUTES

The Greeks often combine fruit and honey. Here we've substituted agave nectar to lighten the glycemic load. Greek yogurt is one of the best new products in the American dairy case—you won't believe how creamy it is.

1 green apple, peeled, cored and diced

1 Anjou pear, peeled, cored and diced

1 firm kiwifruit, peeled and diced

2 tablespoons orange juice

2 teaspoons agave nectar

2 cups nonfat plain Greek yogurt

In a medium bowl, combine the apple, pear, and kiwi. In a small cup, stir the orange juice and agave nectar until combined. Add to the fruit and toss to coat. Refrigerate for at least 30 minutes before serving.

Place 1 cup yogurt in each of 2 serving bowls. Top with the fruit salad and serve.

LUNCH

Quinoa Tabouli with Roasted Sweet Potato

SERVES 2

PREP TIME: 5 MINUTES • COOK TIME: 18 MINUTES

Sweet potatoes are a nutritional powerhouse: low in fat and calories, they deliver huge amounts of vitamins A and C and add a sweet flavor and creamy texture to any dish. No wonder so many cultures include them in their diets!

TIP: Although quinoa is not often used in Greek cuisine, we've used it in this salad because of its protein content. If you can't find quinoa, use couscous.

1 small sweet potato (about 8 ounces), peeled and cut into ½-inch dice

½ teaspoon olive oil

Salt and black pepper

¾ cup quinoa

½ cup white kidney or cannellini beans, drained and rinsed

¼ cup fresh lemon juice

½ cup chopped fresh mint

½ cup chopped fresh parsley

Preheat the oven to 375°F. In an 8-inch square baking dish, toss the sweet potato, oil, and salt and pepper to taste. Roast for 16 to 18 minutes, until tender, stirring often.

Meanwhile, cook the quinoa according to the package directions.

In a serving bowl, combine the sweet potato, beans, cooked quinoa, lemon juice, mint, and parsley. Toss to coat, season with salt and pepper, and serve.

Baked Shrimp and Feta Casserole

SERVES 2

PREP TIME: 5 MINUTES • COOK TIME: 24 MINUTES

Feta, a crumbly cheese made from sheep's or goat's milk, is the cheese used most often in Greek cooking. Its briny flavor means that a little goes a long way.

TIP: Reach for frozen shrimp—it's already cooked and ready to go.

1 teaspoon olive oil

½ small onion, chopped

1 ½ cups cooked brown rice

Salt and black pepper

¾ pound frozen precooked (peeled and deveined) shrimp, thawed

1 can (15 ounces) diced tomatoes, drained

2 tablespoons crumbled reduced-fat feta cheese

2 tablespoons minced fresh dill

Preheat the oven to 350°F. Warm the oil in a medium ovenproof non-stick skillet over medium-low heat. Add the onion; cook for 4 minutes, until softened. Remove from the heat and stir in the rice. Season with salt and pepper.

Arrange the shrimp and tomatoes on top of the rice. Sprinkle with the feta and dill. Bake for 20 minutes, until the shrimp turn pink and are warmed through. Serve.

Greek Salad with Fresh Lemon Dressing

SERVES 2

PREP TIME: 10 MINUTES • COOK TIME: 3 MINUTES

Long a staple of the Greeks, this crispy, crunchy, colorful salad deserves a spot on any dinner table.

TIP: Use extra virgin olive oil in salads and other uncooked dishes. The less expensive regular press olive oil is fine for cooking.

1 tablespoon fresh lemon juice

¼ teaspoon dried oregano, crumbled

1 small clove garlic, minced, plus ½ clove garlic

Salt and black pepper

2 teaspoons extra-virgin olive oil

2 whole-grain pitas

3 cups chopped romaine lettuce

¾ cup cherry or grape tomatoes cut in half

½ small cucumber, peeled, cut in half lengthwise, and thinly sliced crosswise

1 cup canned chickpeas, drained and rinsed

2 tablespoons crumbled reduced-fat feta cheese

In a large serving bowl, whisk the lemon juice, oregano, minced garlic, and salt and pepper to taste. Add the oil and 1 teaspoon water; whisk until well combined.

Heat a grill pan over high heat until smoking; lightly coat with cooking spray. Rub the outsides of the pitas with the garlic half. Grill for 3 minutes, turning often, until grill marks appear but the pitas are not quite crispy.

Add the lettuce, tomatoes, cucumber, chickpeas, and cheese to the dressing; toss to coat. Serve with the warm pitas.

Greek Tuna Melt

SERVES 2

PREP TIME: 5 MINUTES • COOK TIME: 2 MINUTES

The climate of Greece means that tomatoes can be grown throughout much of the year. They make a perfect partner for tuna and salty feta cheese, with pita wedges for scooping.

1 can (6 ounces) solid albacore tuna packed in water, drained and
squeezed dry

1 teaspoon olive oil

1 teaspoon red wine vinegar

Salt and black pepper

1 large tomato, cored and thinly sliced (about 6 slices)

1 ounce reduced-fat feta cheese, crumbled

1 teaspoon chopped fresh oregano

2 whole-grain pitas, cut into wedges

In a small bowl, toss the tuna, oil, vinegar, and salt and pepper to taste.

Arrange the tomato slices, overlapping slightly on a large microwave-safe plate. Top with the tuna mixture and feta. Microwave for 2 minutes, until the cheese bubbles and the tuna is warmed through. Sprinkle with the oregano. Serve hot with the pita wedges.

Tzatziki

MAKES 1½ CUPS

PREP TIME: 5 MINUTES

Tzatziki is a creamy, incredibly versatile dish that's used as a dip, sandwich spread, or sauce. A cousin of India's raita, tzatziki is best made with thick Greek yogurt.

½ cucumber, peeled and seeded

1 small clove garlic, minced

2 teaspoons white wine vinegar

1 teaspoon extra-virgin olive oil

1 ¼ cups nonfat plain Greek yogurt

2 tablespoons chopped fresh mint, dill, or tarragon

Salt

2 whole-grain pitas, cut into wedges

Grate the cucumber onto a cutting board. Wrap in a paper towel and squeeze to soak up the moisture. In a medium bowl, combine the cucumber, garlic, vinegar, and oil. Stir in the yogurt and mint until combined; season with salt. Serve with the pita wedges.

White Bean Salad with Sugar Snap Peas and Tomatoes

SERVES 2

PREP TIME: 5 MINUTES • COOK TIME: 2 MINUTES

Beans are an excellent source of protein, and canned beans are a quick cook's savior for hearty, healthy salads like this one.

TIP: For the brightest flavor and color, fresh herbs are a must in uncooked salads.

4 ounces sugar snap peas

3 tablespoons fresh lemon juice

1 teaspoon extra-virgin olive oil

Salt and black pepper

1 ½ cups canned white kidney or cannellini beans, rinsed

1 cup cherry tomatoes cut in half

1 tablespoon chopped fresh oregano

¼ cup chopped fresh flat-leaf parsley

Spinach or romaine lettuce leaves

Bring a pot of water to a boil. Add the snap peas; cook for 2 minutes, until crisp-tender. Drain.

In a serving bowl, whisk the lemon juice, oil, and salt and pepper to taste. Add the peas, beans, tomatoes, oregano, and parsley. Arrange the spinach leaves on 2 serving plates, top with the salad, and serve.

Chicken and Eggplant Stacks

SERVES 2

PREP TIME: 5 MINUTES • COOK TIME: 22 MINUTES

This clever stack makes a quick and filling snack. Serve with a green salad and Middle Eastern flatbread, if you can find it.

1 boneless, skinless chicken breast half (about 4 ounces)

2 thick slices (about 1/2 inch) eggplant

4 thick slices (about 1/2 inch) tomato

Salt and black pepper

1/4 cup thinly sliced fresh basil leaves

1 ounce shredded part-skim mozzarella cheese

Preheat the oven to 350°F. Lightly coat a medium nonstick skillet with cooking spray; set over medium-high heat. Slice the chicken breast in half horizontally to make two thin fillets. Add the chicken and eggplant to the skillet; cook for 2 minutes per side, until lightly browned. The eggplant will start to soften; the chicken will not be cooked through.

Place the eggplant in a 9-inch baking pan. Top each slice with 1 tomato slice. Sprinkle with salt and pepper to taste and the basil. Place the chicken on top of the vegetables; top with the remaining tomato slices. Season with salt and pepper; sprinkle evenly with the cheese. Bake for 18 minutes, until the chicken is cooked through. Serve.

Grilled Chicken and Tomato Souvlaki

SERVES 2

PREP TIME: 5 MINUTES (PLUS MARINADE)   •   COOK TIME: 7 MINUTES

TIP: If you are using wooden skewers, soak them in water for at least 10 minutes before assembling the kebabs to prevent scorching.

2 tablespoons red wine vinegar

1 teaspoon olive oil

2 teaspoons chopped fresh oregano, or 1 teaspoon dried

Salt and black pepper

12 ounces boneless, skinless chicken breasts, cut into sixteen $3/4$-inch cubes

8 cherry tomatoes

1 zucchini, cut into sixteen 1-inch chunks

In a medium nonreactive bowl, combine the vinegar, oil, oregano, and salt and pepper to taste. Add the chicken and toss to coat. Cover and refrigerate for at least 2 hours.

Preheat the grill or a grill pan over medium-high heat. Using eight 8- to 10-inch skewers, thread 2 pieces of chicken, 1 tomato, and 2 zucchini chunks on each skewer. Grill for 5 to 7 minutes, turning until well browned on all sides. Serve.

DINNER

Homemade Gyros

SERVES 2

PREP TIME: (PLUS MARINADE) • COOK TIME: 10 MINUTES

Gyros are a popular street food in Greece. Think of them as a sandwich, and add your favorite fillings. Here we use tomato, tzatziki, and red onion.

1 teaspoon paprika

1 teaspoon chopped fresh oregano, or ¼ teaspoon dried

Salt and black pepper

1 boneless pork loin (about 12 ounces), thinly sliced

½ teaspoon white wine vinegar

2 whole-grain pitas

¼ cup tzatziki (see recipe page 250)

½ cup thinly sliced red onion

1 tomato, cored and thinly sliced

In a small bowl, combine the paprika, oregano, and salt and pepper to taste.

Using a mallet or the bottom of a heavy saucepan, pound the pork slices to less than ¼ inch thick. Place in a nonreactive 9-by-13-inch pan. Sprinkle with the paprika mixture, then drizzle with the vinegar. Refrigerate for 30 minutes.

Coat a large nonstick skillet with cooking spray; place over high heat. Cook the meat for 3 minutes per side, until browned and cooked through.

Wrap the pitas in foil and warm in the oven. Fill with the pork, tzatziki, onion, and tomato. Serve.

Lemon-Garlic Roasted Cod with Warm Bulgur

SERVES 2

PREP TIME: 5 MINUTES • COOK TIME: 10 MINUTES

Searing the fish before roasting gives it a nice golden crust. Use an oven-proof skillet so that there's only one pan to clean.

TIP: If you can't find bulgur, use brown rice.

1 clove garlic, minced

Salt and black pepper

1 teaspoon olive oil

½ teaspoon finely grated lemon zest

1 tablespoon fresh lemon juice

2 cod fillets (about 5 ounces each)

Warm bulgur with asparagus (see below)

Preheat the oven to 400°F. In small cup, mash the garlic and salt to taste to form a paste. Stir in the oil, lemon zest, and lemon juice.

Lightly coat a medium ovenproof nonstick skillet with cooking spray; place over medium-high heat. Season the cod with salt and pepper to taste. Add to the hot pan; cook for 2 minutes per side, until lightly browned. The fish will not be cooked through. Spread the garlic mixture over the fish. Transfer the skillet to the oven; roast the fish for 6 minutes, until opaque in the center. Serve the bulgur on top.

Warm Bulgur with Asparagus: Cook ½ cup bulgur according to the package directions. Add 1 cup chopped asparagus in the last 3 minutes of cooking. Drain. In a medium bowl, whisk 2 teaspoons fresh lemon juice, 1 teaspoon olive oil, and salt and pepper to taste. Toss the bulgur and asparagus with the dressing. Toss in ½ cup chopped fresh parsley or basil.

PART 5

THE 5-FACTOR WORLD DIET MENUS

Now that you've pored over all the recipes, you can start designing your daily menus. Here I provide four weeks of sample menus, including snacks. Each week is designed to create the perfect mix of cholesterol-lowering, cancer-fighting meals. This four-week plan also incorporates some aspects of my proven 5-Factor weight-loss formula for even greater fitness results.

WEEK 1

DAY 1	DAY 2	DAY 3
Breakfast: Miso Soup with Tofu	**Breakfast:** Smooth Peach-Raspberry Lassi	**Breakfast:** Crisp Scallion and Rice Omelet
Snack 1: Crostini Caprese	**Snack 1:** Creamy Apple, Celery, and Red Onion Salad	**Snack 1:** Indian-Spiced Chickpea and Chicken Bowl
Lunch: Quinoa Tabouli with Roasted Sweet Potato	**Lunch:** Easy Niçoise Salad	**Lunch:** Whole Wheat Pasta with Basil and Spinach Pesto
Snack 2: Charred Sweet Peppers with Ricotta	**Snack 2:** Golden Split Pea Soup	**Snack 2:** Warm Lavash with Sun-Dried Tomatoes and Creamy Herb Spread
Dinner: Lemon-Garlic Roasted Cod with Warm Bulgur	**Dinner:** Italian Chicken with Peppers and Onions	**Dinner:** Five-Spice Halibut
Activity: Skip the elevator at work; take the stairs instead.	**Activity:** Park in the most remote corner of the lot.	**Activity:** Vacuum the house, even if it's already clean.

DAY 4	DAY 5	DAY 6
Breakfast: Morning Muesli and Hot Coffee	**Breakfast:** Asparagus Mini-Soufflés with Chives	**Breakfast:** Italian Frittata with Zucchini, Leeks, and Parmesan
Snack 1: Smoked Salmon Nori Roll	**Snack 1:** Ginger Chicken Lettuce Wrap	**Snack 1:** Lemon and Parsley Hummus
Lunch: Cool Lemongrass Chicken and Rice Salad	**Lunch:** Soba Noodle Stir-Fry	**Lunch:** Southeast Asian Shrimp Salad
Snack 2: Eggplant Caponata	**Snack 2:** Smoked Salmon Smorgasbord	**Snack 2:** Warm Lentils with Goat Cheese
Dinner: Grilled Sesame-Orange Tuna	**Dinner:** Korean Beef Grill	**Dinner:** Grilled Lemon Chicken with Spiced Couscous
Activity: Out of milk? Walk to the nearest convenience store for a refill.	**Activity:** Even if you're already done shopping, take an extra loop around the mall.	**Activity:** Skip the moving sidewalks at the airport and walk to your gate.

DAY 7: Free Day

WEEK 2

DAY 1	DAY 2	DAY 3
Breakfast: Gaeran Mari	**Breakfast:** Yogurt with Apricot and Pomegranate	**Breakfast:** Fresh Fruit Salad with Yogurt
Snack 1: Balsamic Roasted Tomato and Goat Cheese Crisps	**Snack 1:** Charred Sweet Peppers with Ricotta	**Snack 1:** Peanut Noodles
Lunch: Fresh Herb Falafel	**Lunch:** Oven-Baked Swedish Meatballs	**Lunch:** Chow Mein for Two
Snack 2: Iced Raspberry Green Tea	**Snack 2:** Shrimp and Bok Choy Pot Stickers	**Snack 2:** Shrimp and Black Bean Fried Rice
Dinner: Seared Striped Bass with Fennel and Orange Salad	**Dinner:** Poached Salmon with Herbed Mayonnaise	**Dinner:** Lemon-Caper Braised Halibut
Activity: While chatting on the phone, get up and pace the floor.	**Activity:** Instead of sending an e-mail to your colleague, walk across the office and have the conversation in person.	**Activity:** Take your dog for an extra-long walk. If you don't have a dog, volunteer to walk a neighbor's.

DAY 4	DAY 5	DAY 6
Breakfast: Whole Wheat Crêpes with Fresh Raspberries	**Breakfast:** Spinach Omelet with Two Cheeses	**Breakfast:** Warm Pita with Yogurt and Dill
Snack 1: Warm Lavash with Sun-Dried Tomatoes and Creamy Herb Spread	**Snack 1:** Crisp Vegetable Salad	**Snack 1:** Stuffed Portobello Mushrooms
Lunch: Baked Shrimp and Feta Casserole	**Lunch:** Warm Lentils with Goat Cheese	**Lunch:** Pan Bagna
Snack 2: Fresh Vegetable Hand Roll	**Snack 2:** Chicken and Eggplant Stacks	**Snack 2:** Golden Split Pea Soup
Dinner: Homemade Gyros	**Dinner:** Roasted Pork Tenderloin with Apples	**Dinner:** Spicy Red-Stewed Salmon with Brown Rice
Activity: Carpool! Walk to your neighbor's house in the morning and ride together to work.	**Activity:** If possible, take public transportation.	**Activity:** Go outside and garden.

DAY 7: Free Day

WEEK 3

DAY 1	DAY 2	DAY 3
Breakfast: Orange-Almond Biscotti with Caffè Latte	**Breakfast:** Swedish Pancakes with Raspberries	**Breakfast:** Spiced Rice Congee with Pear
Snack 1: Three-Pea Stir-Fry	**Snack 1:** Greek Tuna Melt	**Snack 1:** Eggplant Caponata
Lunch: Creamed Herring on Brown Bread	**Lunch:** Egg Drop Soup with Fresh Spinach	**Lunch:** Roasted Tomato Quinoa with Fresh Herbs and Thick Yogurt
Snack 2: Tzatziki	**Snack 2:** Open-Faced Chicken and Caramelized Onion Sandwich	**Snack 2:** Shrimp and Noodle Stir-Fry
Dinner: Salmon Teriyaki with Asian Coleslaw	**Dinner:** Shabu-Shabu	**Dinner:** Moules Marinades

DAY 4	DAY 5	DAY 6
Breakfast: Chicken Noodle Soup	**Breakfast:** Warm Cinnamon Bulgur with Nuts and Berries	**Breakfast:** Crunchy Toasted Granola
Snack 1: Spicy Tuna Sushi Roll	**Snack 1:** Chicken and Eggplant Stacks	**Snack 1:** Curried Chicken Wontons
Lunch: BBQ Beef Rice Bowl	**Lunch:** Greek Salad with Fresh Lemon Dressing	**Lunch:** Soupe au Pistou
Snack 2: Pickled Cucumber with Fresh Dill on Rye Crisps	**Snack 2:** Roasted Asparagus with Quinoa and Parmesan Curls	**Snack 2:** Fresh Vegetable Hand Roll
Dinner: Garlic Chicken Cassoulet	**Dinner:** Seared Sesame Scallops in Noodle Broth	**Dinner:** Lamb and Tomato Stew

DAY 7: Free Day

WEEK 4

DAY 1	DAY 2	DAY 3
Breakfast: Curried Sweet Potato with Warm Paratha Bread	**Breakfast:** Soba Noodle Bowl with Cucumber and Cabbage	**Breakfast:** Sesame Rice Bowl
Snack 1: Seaweed Salad with Edamame	**Snack 1:** White Bean Salad with Sugar Snap Peas and Tomatoes	**Snack 1:** Roasted Garlic Baba Ghanoush
Lunch: Crispy Spiced Chicken	**Lunch:** Spicy Lamb and Feta Pita Pizzas	**Lunch:** Sweet Potato Risotto with Veal Cutlets
Snack 2: Warm Ratatouille	**Snack 2:** Pork and Cabbage Dumplings	**Snack 2:** Chicken Yakatori
Dinner: Spicy Beef Stir-Fry with Black Bean Sauce	**Dinner:** Pronto Chicken with Porcini Ragù	**Dinner:** Classic Home-Style Korean Stir-Fry

DAY 4	DAY 5	DAY 6
Breakfast: Coconut Spinach Cup	**Breakfast:** Miso Soup with Tofu	**Breakfast:** Italian Frittata with Zucchini, Leeks, and Parmesan
Snack 1: Smoked Trout and Horseradish Cream Open-Faced Sandwich	**Snack 1:** Grilled Chicken and Tomato Souvlaki	**Snack 1:** Sautéed Shallot Spinach with Brown Rice
Lunch: Mee Goreng (Singapore Noodle)	**Lunch:** Fried Rice with Mushrooms and Edamame	**Lunch:** Southeast Asian Shrimp Salad
Snack 2: Spicy Dahl	**Snack 2:** Blueberry Rye Muffins	**Snack 2:** Smoked Salmon Smorgasbord
Dinner: Ginger Beef and Noodles	**Dinner:** Tandoori Chicken with Cool Raita	**Dinner:** Chicken and Sweet Potato Stir-Fry

DAY 7: Free Day

Shopping Suggestions

STORES

Cost Plus World Market (www.worldmarket.com): World Market is an unbeatable resource for foods from all over the world. Go there for herring and smoked salmon if you're craving Scandinavian, vinegars and olive oils if you prefer Mediterranean, or an assortment of sauces if you want to go Asian. There are stores all over the United States, except in the Northeast.

Trader Joe's (www.traderjoes.com): Trader Joe's offers economical shopping options for World Dieters. With most foods made under the company's own label, Trader Joe's focuses on all-natural, heart-healthy goods. You can see the influences of many different countries' culinary traditions as you browse the store. There are Trader Joe's stores up and down both coasts and quite a few in the Midwest as well.

Whole Foods Market (www.wholefoodsmarket.com): Whole Foods is a must-visit grocery store for anyone opting to go international. You can find crackers, snacks, sauces, and seaweeds in every aisle of the country's biggest natural market. The prepared-foods section of Whole Foods usually has a great selection of fresh sushi, sesame tofu, and other healthy items to go. Whole Foods stores are scattered across the country.

Other Chains: Safeway (www.safeway.com) and other national grocery chains almost always have an international aisle, so no matter where you live, you will probably be able to find reduced-sodium soy sauce, smoked salmon, various legumes, and other World Diet essentials—usually for an impressively low price. At your local store, ask to be directed to the international section. You might be surprised by the selection that awaits you.

ONLINE OPTIONS

You can often get great deals shopping online, especially if you're buying in bulk. Here are a few sites worth considering:

General

EthnicFoodsCo.com (www.ethnicfoodsco.com): EthnicFoodsCo.com is an excellent one-stop-shopping destination for the World Dieter. The website is broken down by country, with "stores" for Greek, Japanese, Chinese, Middle Eastern, Thai, and Indian foods. This website also sells innovative "food baskets" with all the ingredients you need to prepare a meal for four. The Chinese basket, for example, includes fried rice seasoning, jasmine rice, braising sauce, noodle soup, Szechuan chili paste, and a choice of appetizers and desserts. It's perfect for someone just launching an international kitchen!

EthnicGrocer.com (www.ethnicgrocer.com): Here you can stock up on the basics. The website is organized by country, so you can choose "pantry essentials" from a huge number of countries, including Spain, China, France, Greece, Italy, Japan, and Korea. This online grocer stocks breads, cereals, snacks, olives, pastas and noodles, sauces, chiles and other peppers, vinegars and cooking oils, soups and broths, and seasonings galore. If you can name it, chances are EthnicGrocer.com has it.

GourmetFoodMall.com (www.gourmetfoodmall.com): GourmetFood Mall.com is a wonderful resource with an ever-expanding menu of food selections from every corner of the planet. You can get everything from sauces to seafood, and you never have to pay for shipping.

Asia

Asian Food Grocer (www.asianfoodgrocer.com): I definitely recommend that you check out Asian Food Grocer, which has everything you could possibly need to start cooking Asian: miso paste, sushi-making sets, a variety of sauces, a huge selection of Asian noodles and teas, wasabi paste, reduced-sodium soy sauce, all kinds of rice (short-grain, Japanese and Chinese, enriched, jasmine, brown), sesame oil, chili sauce, fish sauce, Japanese curry, dashi, and much, much more.

eFoodDepot.com (www.efooddepot.com): eFoodDepot.com doesn't just sell Asian food, although it does specialize in items imported from China, Japan, Thailand, India, and Indonesia. You can also find a wide array of foods from Europe, South America, and the Middle East. The prices are extremely competitive, too.

EverythingChopsticks.com (www.everythingchopsticks.com): Getting into the swing of using chopsticks? If so, why not fill your silverware drawer with some sets for everyday use? EverythingChopsticks.com is the best online retailer for this purpose. You can buy everything from plain, daily-use chopsticks to beautiful gift sets for special occasions. The chopsticks, which range in price from just over $1 a pair to more than $25 a pair, come in all sorts of materials—lacquered, wooden, steel, and bamboo—so you might want to experiment and see which type suits you best. You can even buy colorful chopsticks made just for kids.

KoaMart.com (www.koamart.com): KoaMart.com sells udon noodles, seaweed, chili paste, premade kimchi dishes, tofu, and some organic foods. This affordable website even sells instant Korean porridge.

Northern Europe

igourmet.com (www.igourmet.com): This is a wonderful website specializing in upscale French products such as cheeses and olive oils. It can be a little pricey, but if you're looking for the perfect French touch to your cooking—such as fleur de sel—igourmet.com is a reliable source. You can also find foods from Italy, India, Sweden, Spain, and many other countries.

Meijer Grocery Express (www.meijergroceryexpress.com): The grocery arm of the retail chain Meijer sells a small selection of Swedish and Scandinavian foods, most notably lingonberries, muesli, and Swedish crispbread.

Saveur du Jour (www.saveurdujour.com): This is the online store for the real Francophile. The mouthwatering selection of French foods—mustards, *herbes de Provence*, honeys, jams, and olive oils—will keep you busy in the kitchen for months.

Mediterranean and Middle East

AmigoFoods.com (www.amigofoods.com): AmigoFoods.com sells items from Spain and Latin America. Choose from beverages, condiments, paella mixes, even sausages and cheeses.

Dayna's Market (www.daynasmarket.com): Dayna's specializes in Mediterranean foods. Browse the market's website for good deals on pita bread, spices, olive oils, bulgur, tahini, nuts, and seeds.

EuropeGourmet.com (www.europegourmet.com): If you're looking for some Spanish specialties, EuropeGourmet.com is a good place to start. You can get everything from typical Spanish spices to extremely expensive Spanish hams.

International Foods (www.oliveimports.com): This is a great place to find Greek and other Mediterranean foods on the Web. It has a good selection of olives, condiments, olive oils, artichokes, roasted red peppers, and other Mediterranean staples.

La Tienda (www.tienda.com): The motto of this online retailer is "the best of Spain" and the website fulfills its promise. With hams, chorizos, and an assortment of typical Spanish spices such as saffron, La Tienda is a great resource for any aspiring Iberian chefs.

Shamra.com (www.shamra.com): Shamra.com sells all sorts of food from the Mediterranean region and Middle East—everything from grape leaves to dried lentils and rice. You can also choose from a number of different tahini pastes if you decide to make your own hummus at home.

Zamouri Spices (www.zamourispices.com): Zamouri Spices is the place to go if you want to get serious about spices. It stocks a huge assortment of Middle Eastern spices and spice blends, plus coffees, teas, and even a line of Moorish beauty products.

Notes

INTRODUCTION

1 World Health Organization, "Obesity and Overweight" (Fact Sheet No. 311, September 2006).

CHAPTER 1: THE WORLD'S FATTEST PEOPLE

1. World Health Organization, "Obesity and Overweight" (Fact Sheet No. 311, September 2006).
2. Phil Mercer, "South Pacific Is Fattest Region," BBC News, bbc.co.uk/z/hi/health/6396111.stm, February 26, 2007; "World's Fattest Countries," *Forbes,* www.forbes.com/2007/02/07/worlds-fattest-countries-forbeslife.cx-ls-0208 worldfat.html, February 7, 2007.
3. National Center for Health Statistics, "Prevalence of Overweight and Obesity Among Adults: United States, 1999–2002," September 9, 2008, http://www.cdc.gov/nchs/products/pubs/pubd/hestats/obese/obse99.htm.
4. National Institutes of Health, "NIH Releases Research Strategy to Fight Obesity Epidemic," August 24, 2004, http://www.nih.gov/news/pr/aug2004/niddk-24.htm.
5. U.S. Department of Health and Human Services, Centers for Disease Control

and Prevention, "Preventing Obesity and Chronic Diseases Through Good Nutrition and Physical Activity," August 2008.

6. "Welcome to the Town That Will Help You Lose Weight," *The Times* (London), February 18, 2007.

7. "You Want Fries with That?" *The New York Times,* January 12, 2003.

8. "Study Details 30-Year Increase in Calorie Consumption," *The New York Times*, February 6, 2004.

9. "Portion Sizes Grow with American Waistlines," Associated Press, December 6, 2006, http://www.msnbc.msn.com/id/16076842/ns/health-diet-and-nutrition/.

10. "Are We Eating Too Much at Restaurants?" *Argus Leader* (Sioux Falls, SD), June 18, 2006.

11. "Size Can Fool the Eyes: Larger Dishes Can Make It Difficult to Limit Your Portions," *The News-Sentinel* (Fort Wayne, IN), November 25, 2008.

12. McDonald's, "Our Story" (FAQ), http://www.mcdonalds.ca/en/aboutus/faq .aspx, accessed May 21, 2009.

13. "A Global Response to a Global Problem: The Epidemic of Overnutrition," *Bulletin of the World Health Organization* 80, no. 12 (2002): 952–8.

14. U.S. Department of Agriculture, "Profiling Food Consumption in America," in *Agricultural Fact Book, 2001–2002* (Washington, DC: Government Printing Office, 2003).

15. "Pedometer Gets People Up and Walking," *The Star-Ledger* (Newark, NJ), November 27, 2007.

16. David Bassett, Jr., et al., "Walking, Cycling, and Obesity Rates in Europe, North America, and Australia," *Journal of Physical Activity and Health* 5 (November 2008): 807.

CHAPTER 2: THE WORLD'S HEALTHIEST PEOPLE

1. CIA, *The 2007 World Factbook*.

2. U.S. Census Bureau, "Income Climbs, Poverty Stabilizes, Uninsured Rate Increases" (press release, August 29, 2006).

3. "Infant Mortality Rates Are Rising in U.S., While Rates in Other Countries Are Improving," ABC News, November 1, 2005.

CHAPTER 3: JAPAN

1. For each country, the sources are the same.
Average life expectancy: CIA, *The 2009 World Factbook*, estimate.
Percentage of overweight/obese adults: World Health Organization, Global InfoBase, http://apps.who.int/infobase/report.aspx.
Meat consumption: World Resources Institute, http://www.wri.org. Diet composition: tk

2. "Percentage of Japanese Aged 65 or Older Hits New High," Associated Press Worldstream, September 17, 2007.

3. World Health Organization, Regional Office for the Western Pacific, "Smok-

ing Statistics" (fact sheets, May 28, 2002); "Death Be Not Proud," *The Economist,* May 1, 2008.

4. "The Secret of Life: Okinawans, The World's Longest-Lived People, Have a Lot to Teach Americans on the Art of Reaching 100," *The Boston Globe,* May 22, 2001.

5. "Smaller Portions Keep Japanese Fit and Trim," *Orlando Sentinel* (Orlando, FL), September 25, 2007.

6. Asian Food Information Centre, "It's a Small World After All: Dietary Guidelines Around the World," 2004.

7. "Simple Living in Japan: Profile," *National Geographic,* http://www.national geographic.com/healthyliving/index.html.

8. David Bassett, Jr., et al., "Walking, Cycling, and Obesity Rates in Europe, North America, and Australia," *Journal of Physical Activity and Health* 5 (November 2008): 809.

CHAPTER 5: CHINA

1. World Health Organization, Regional Office for the Western Pacific, "Smoking Statistics" (fact sheet, May 28, 2002).

2. T. Colin Campbell with Thomas M. Campbell II, *The China Study: The Most Comprehensive Study of Nutrition Ever Conducted* (Dallas, Tx: BenBella Books, 2004), 90.

3. Ibid., 78.

4. Ibid., 82, 86.

5. Tea Association of the U.S.A., "About Tea," http://www.teausa.com/general/501g.cfm.

6. Mary Jo Manzanares, "Help! I'm a Prisoner in a Chinese Fortune Cookie Factory," Fly Away Cafe, BlissTree.com, April 10, 2007.

7. "Wok Carefully: CSPI Takes a (Second) Look at Chinese Restaurant Food," Center for Science March 21, 2007, cspinet.org/new/200703211.html/.

8. *Irish Independent*, "How the French Really Have Their Gateau and Eat it." February 28, 2008.

CHAPTER 6: SWEDEN

1. "World's Healthiest Countries," *Foreign Policy,* October 2007.

CHAPTER 7: FRANCE

1. "7 Secret Ways French Women Stay Slim," *Cosmopolitan,* February 2003.

CHAPTER 8: ITALY

1. Organisation for Economic Co-operation and Development, Health Data 2008, "How Does Italy Compare."

2. "The Hidden Calories in Your Drinks," ABC News, January 23, 2005.
3. K. Maruyama et al., "The Joint Impact on Being Overweight of Self Reported Behaviours of Eating Quickly and Eating Until Full: Cross Sectional Survey," *British Medical Journal* (October 21, 2008): 337.

CHAPTER 9: SPAIN

1. J-P Chaput et al., "Relationship Between Short Sleeping Hours and Childhood Overweight/Obesity: Results from the 'Québec en Forme' Project," *International Journal of Obesity* 30 (March 14, 2006): 1080–85.
2. "Suburban Sprawl Adds Health Concern," *The New York Times,* August 31, 2003.

CHAPTER 10: SOUTH KOREA

1. "Uniqueness of Korean Cuisine: Kimchi," *Korea Times,* July 31, 2008.
2. U.S. Department of Agriculture, Economic Research Service, "Factors Affecting U.S. Beef Consumption" (Outlook Report No. LDPM13502, October 2005).

CHAPTER 11: ISRAEL

1. "Common Indian Spice Stirs Hope," *The Wall Street Journal*, TK.

CHAPTER 12: GREECE

1. "Dueling Diets," *Harvard Public Health Review*, Fall 2004.
2. "Study Highlights Unhealthy Eating Habits Among Greek Children," Athens News Agency, November 13, 2007.

CHAPTER 16: THE 5-FACTOR LIFESTYLE

1. David Bassett, Jr., et al., "Walking, Cycling, and Obesity Rates in Europe, North America, and Australia," *Journal of Physical Activity and Health* 5 (November 2008): 795–814.
2. "Pedometers Help People Stay Active, Stanford Study Finds," Stanford School of Medicine, November 26, 2007.
3. I. M. Lee et al., "Physical Activity and Coronary Heart Disease in Women: Is 'No Pain, No Gain' Passé?" *Journal of the American Medical Association* 285, no. 11 (March 21, 2001): 1447–54.

Index

Recipe Index

Acknowledgments

I Would Like to Thank:

My Canadian parents, who instilled in me my love for travel and the spirit of adventure.

My Hungarian, Polish, and Romanian grandparents, and my Cuban and Israeli cousins.

My American, Brazilian, Mexican, Canadian, French, English, Swiss, Italian, Greek, Irish, Portuguese, German, Chinese, Spanish, Australian, Iranian, Dominican, and Bahamian clients, for bringing me along on their journeys and entrusting me with their health.

My British/French business right hand, Alex Nesbitt, for being the CPU for everything I do.

Canada, the most multicultural country in the world, and Toronto, the most ethnically diverse city in the world. Thank you for inspiring me.

My American superagent, Andrea Barzvi.

Laura Moser. Thank you for turning my incoherent ramblings into beautiful, articulate chapters.

Susie Ott, for helping me create 5-Factor–friendly recipes that taste delicious with ingredients I've never heard of.

My editor, Marnie Cochran. I waited six years to work with you!

Nancy, Steve, and Holly, for making my abstract ideas physical objects that people enjoy.

My lawyer, Wendy Heller, for being tough so I don't have to be.

New Balance, for making sure my feet are comfortable while I run around the world, and FUZE, for keeping me hydrated during all my travels.

ABOUT THE AUTHOR

HARLEY PASTERNAK, M.Sc., is a *New York Times* bestselling author and holds a master's of science in exercise physiology and nutritional sciences from the University of Toronto, as well as an honors degree in kinesiology from the University of Western Ontario. He is certified by the American College of Sports Medicine and the Canadian Society for Exercise Physiology. He has appeared on *The Oprah Winfrey Show, Today,* CNN, *America's Next Top Model, Rachael Ray,* and *Tyra*. Pasternak lives and works in Los Angeles.

www.harleypasternak.com
www.5factorworlddiet.com